CORPORATIZING AMERICAN HEALTH CARE

CORPORATIZING AMERICAN HEALTH CARE

How We Lost Our Health Care System

ROBERT W. DERLET, MD

JOHNS HOPKINS UNIVERSITY PRESS | *Baltimore*

© 2021 Johns Hopkins University Press
All rights reserved. Published 2021
Printed in the United States of America on acid-free paper
9 8 7 6 5 4 3 2 1

Johns Hopkins University Press
2715 North Charles Street
Baltimore, Maryland 21218-4363
www.press.jhu.edu

Library of Congress Cataloging-in-Publication Data

Names: Derlet, Robert W., 1949– author.
Title: Corporatizing American health care : how we lost our health care system /
   Robert W. Derlet, MD.
Description: Baltimore : Johns Hopkins University Press, [2021] |
   Includes bibliographical references and index.
Identifiers: LCCN 2020009008 | ISBN 9781421439587 (paperback ; alk. paper) |
   ISBN 9781421439594 (ebook)
Subjects: MESH: Delivery of Health Care—economics | Health Care Sector—
   economics | Insurance, Health—economics | Health Care Reform | Politics |
   Health Policy | United States
Classification: LCC R728 | NLM W 84 AA1 | DDC 338.4/73621—dc23
LC record available at https://lccn.loc.gov/2020009008

A catalog record for this book is available from the British Library.

*Special discounts are available for bulk purchases of this book. For more information,
please contact Special Sales at specialsales@press.jhu.edu.*

Johns Hopkins University Press uses environmentally friendly book materials,
including recycled text paper that is composed of at least 30 percent post-consumer
waste, whenever possible.

CONTENTS

Just after the fall of the Iron Curtain in the 1990s, I was invited to the former Soviet Republic of Belarus (White Russia) as a visiting professor. The day before I departed from the United States, I had dinner at a small "mom and pop" diner in California. The waitress was all smiles, quickly took my order, and handed it to the owner-chef, who produced a delightful and delicious meal in just a few minutes, served hot by the same smiling waitress. "Great service," I thought to myself, and since I have freedom of choice I will come back, once I return home.

A few days later, and almost halfway around the world, I had dinner at a Stalinist hotel, in Minsk, Belarus. After a long wait, a stern-faced waitress took my order. She then walked the order over to an unhappy-appearing official at a nearby desk, who then marched back to my table to ask me my name. He left my table and disappeared behind a squeaky old wooden door. After some minutes, he reappeared and placed my order in a pile at the corner of his desk. Half an hour passed before my waitress picked up my order and took it to another official sitting in the far corner of the restaurant. He let it lay on his desk several minutes, then finally picked it up, compared it to a list he held in his left hand, and then placed check marks on my order. He finally dropped it in a box beside his desk.

After a quarter of an hour, my waitress picked up my order again and handed it to a third official who threw it down on a pile of other papers on his desk. After some moments, he placed numbers by each of the items on my order and added them up with a mechanical adding machine. He then placed my order on the left side of his desk, which was eventually picked up by my waitress and taken back through a squeaky revolving door to the kitchen. Finally, after nearly two and a half hours, I was served my dinner—cold.

But the story does not end there. Near the end of my meal, and after waving my hand like I was flagging down an old Soviet tank, I ordered a cup of coffee from a different annoyed waitress. She told me I needed a special coupon to order coffee, and I had to go to the hotel front desk to get it, which I did. On returning, I handed the coupon to her as she was standing at the kitchen door and, finally, after a long wait received my lukewarm coffee.

So what does my restaurant experience have to do with this book on the evolution of American health care from bedside medicine to corporate medicine? A lot. The efficient American health care system of past years has now evolved into a complex maze of monopolies and a racket of multiple bureaucratic checks, approvals, denials, roadblocks, and detours. The result is a massive and at times redundant workforce that frustrates patients, physicians, nurses, and office staff. Foremost, this complexity allows corporations to siphon off huge profits. Imagine Wall Street taking several dollars at each step of my dinner order. Inefficiency and the drive to generate dollars explain in part why American health care costs are twice as much as in modern European countries.

As a practicing physician, on the front lines of health care for more than 30 years, I have witnessed the transition in the delivery of medical care. The focus has changed from serving the needs of people to generating money. Wall Street has taken notice of the trillions of dollars in the bloodstream of health care. The corporate invasion into this system has opened the door to greed, corruption, and fraud, which has robbed the American people and driven so many into hardship. As a candidate for the US Congress in 2016, I also learned firsthand about the influence corporations hold over Congress, and the frustrations ordinary Americans have about our current health care system.

This book is written to stimulate discussions in the health care policy, economics, and law classes I teach at colleges and universities. I will provide you with a front-seat view into the step-by-step evolution of medical care from an individualized small cottage profession to a giant impersonal corporate industry that costs Americans more than $4 trillion each year. This book is not intended to be a complete analysis of our health care system—that would require a lengthy series of books.

I want to thank my sister Marian Derlet and my colleague Professor Charles Goldman for their encouragement and ongoing moral support to write this book. Two colleagues helped me with initial edits of selected chapters, Paolo Maffei and Sharon Marovich, for which I am grateful.

Our health care system is complex and can be confusing. Sorting through and describing the many multifaceted issues was only possible with the assistance of others. I thank my patients who were willing to share their experiences in the health care system. I also acknowledge the hard work of dedicated nurses, medical assistants, and health care support staff, who advocate what is best for patients. Many physicians shared their experiences, some historic, some contemporary, with me. Most notable include in alphabetical order: Dr. Gene Allred, Dr. Garry Chang, Dr. John Daley, Dr. Nayvin Gordon, Dr. James Hongola, Dr. Edward Panacek, Dr. Arlene Kirschner-Poe, Dr. Ralph Retherford, Dr. John Richards, and Dr. David Suchard. Numerous other individuals provided history, experiences, data, perspective, opinions, and case examples that have helped form the backbone of this book. I thank them but keep their names in confidence. My students in health care classes have helped me better focus and explain the complexities and misconceptions in our health care system.

Perspective on European health care systems was enhanced through discussions with numerous local residents and health care professionals. I specifically want to thank the following professionals: Dr. Anna-Lena Noponen (Finland), Dr. Jouni Kurola (Finland), Dr. Aris Exadaktylos (Switzerland), Dr. Christien van der Linden (Netherlands), Frans de Voeght (Netherlands), Dr. Jana Seblova (Czech Republic), and Dr. Jacques Levraut (France).

And, finally, Dr. Robert McNamara, professor at Temple University in Philadelphia, deserves a big thank you. Many years ago he rang the alarm bells warning of the corporate intrusion into the practice of medicine and stands as a brave pioneer who predicted the impending changes in American health care.

CORPORATIZING AMERICAN HEALTH CARE

The Outrageous Cost of American Health Care

When I first began medical school in San Francisco in the fall of 1971, I had little knowledge about how much money doctors made. I did not know anything about hospital charges, billing policies, or actual costs for services. Nor did any of my classmates understand these or other costs, such as laboratory work, x-rays, surgery, or prescription medications. Like all of my 136 classmates at the University of California, San Francisco (UCSF), we wanted to become doctors to help people, to improve the health of both individuals and their communities, and to have the ability to put to practical use the scientific knowledge we had acquired during our 16 years of education, from elementary school through college. Perhaps we were not taught about health care costs because, relatively speaking, health care was much less expensive then.

My first introduction to the world of health care costs came during my first-year clerkship at Mount Zion Hospital, one of UCSF's many San Francisco teaching hospitals. As medical students, we practiced taking histories and examining patients, which was fun, but then we had the not-so-fun burden of writing about our patient encounters in a document called the "history and physical," known as an H&P. This document written in long hand usually took 10 to 12 pages of ink scrawled onto college-ruled hospital notepaper.

While examining a 60-year-old woman who was scheduled for gall-bladder surgery, I noticed a healing wound on her nose. She told me that a basal cell carcinoma of the skin had been removed a week earlier. I asked how much the procedure had cost, and she told me $50 ($260 in today's dollars), which she paid for with cash. But I was less interested in the cost and more excited when my preceptor let me take out the 10 stitches that had been used to close her surgical wound.

Fast-forward to 2018. I was working in a small rural clinic in the Sierra Nevada foothills of California. On a cold wintry day, I was running late because many of my patients had difficulty getting to the clinic because of an unexpected heavy snowfall. In midafternoon, I examined a 60-year-old woman who had waited patiently to have the new skin growth on her nose examined. Her skin growth looked just like a basal cell carcinoma, and I referred her to an out-of-town dermatologist for a biopsy and, most likely, surgery. Over the next several weeks, she made many trips to the skin specialist. She agreed to have the growth surgically removed only after checking and rechecking with her health care insurance company that the dermatologist was in network. After she had the in-office surgical procedure, she received a bill from the doctor for $6,000. Her insurance company refused to pay because, it turned out, the dermatologist was out of network. How did we get from $50 to $6,000 for the same procedure, the same cancer, on the same side of the nose? And, then, how is it that a health care insurance plan could refuse to pay for cancer treatment?

Health care costs have grown exponentially in my lifetime. Health care expenditures in America approached $4 trillion in 2020, and consume over 18% of the US gross domestic product. That's more than $12,000 for each person in this country each year. And that sum is two times what it costs in most Western European countries to deliver care to their people. In Europe, the population as a whole receives equal or even better health care for close to $6,000 per year per person on average.

Over the past 50 years, health care costs have grown from an afterthought for many families, with nearly all costs paid for by a health care plan, to the topic of dinner-table conversation and one of the top worries of American families today. Many of my patients have shared their horror stories about the health care system, and I have included many of these stories throughout this book.

The current cost of health care in America is outrageous. In 2010, the Affordable Care Act (ACA) was passed and signed into law by President Barack Obama. One of the compelling reasons for this new federal law was the disgraceful and unaffordable cost of health care. The ACA may have slowed the growth of this monster industry, but only by a little. Managers of Wall Street hedge funds have quickly learned the loopholes that allow them to siphon off our hard-earned dollars for profit and administrative waste, money that should be used for actual hands-on health care.

Our health care delivery system is sometimes referred to as the *health care industrial complex*. It is like a gigantic, business-oriented octopus, reaching out to take large chunks of hard-earned money out of our wallets. While prices skyrocket, our politicians in Washington, DC, argue about how to fix it and, at the same time, provide loopholes to an industry that allows it to legally cheat us. Both Republicans and Democrats welcome industry lobbyists into their offices as well as huge political contributions from pharmaceutical, hospital, insurance, and physician groups, as described in a *Washington Post* article (Stein and Abutaleb 2019): "This week, pharmaceutical companies, hospitals, insurance companies and medical device manufacturers practically ran the table in Congress, winning hundreds of billions of dollars in tax breaks and other gifts through old-fashioned lobbying, re-exerting their political prowess." Lobbying and campaign contributions result in regulations that guarantee these groups billions of dollars in excessive profits and, in the end, make the average American family pay.

Who Makes the Rules?

During the 2018 election cycle, Senator Mitch McConnell (R-KY), the Senate Majority leader, received campaign contributions of over $150,000 from pharmaceutical groups, and Senator Sherrod Brown

(D-OH) received over $250,000 from hospital groups. It adds up when all 535 members of Congress are included; insurance groups in 2018 alone spent $180,000,000 in combined lobbying and campaign contributions. And hospital organizations have spent nearly a billion dollars on lobbying the US Congress over the past 10 years—to suck more money from you. With such money spent on Congress to increase the money flow in health care, is it any surprise that our health care costs are outrageous?

The driving forces that result in outrageous health care costs in America can only be solved by legislation by the US Congress.

Doctors, the majority of whom attended medical school to help humanity, now find themselves stuck in the middle as pawns in a complex health delivery system. Doctors (and mid-level practitioners) order drugs, laboratory tests, x-ray imaging, MRIs, surgery, hospitalization, and so on. These things all make money for pharmaceutical companies, hospitals, other physicians, supply companies, limited liability corporations, and large interstate conglomerates. Without the "doctors order," there is little or no money for these profit-making entities. But, even now, few medical schools and teaching hospitals spend much time teaching students about health care costs and the power and control that they will have as individual physicians.

Shall we return to the horse-and-buggy days of health care? Absolutely not. Medical care has made tremendous advances over the past 30 years—better medications, incredible cancer cures, and new space-age surgical techniques. But these advances should not quadruple health care costs. Much of the increased costs to Americans is caused by Wall Street business models and mindsets that seek to maximize profits. I have personally observed that the European systems of health care are just as advanced as our health care and provide it at 50% of the amount we spend (see chapter 5).

So what happened? Why does health care cost far more now than when I began my career? Why do families worry about bankruptcy and homelessness because of unaffordable hospital bills? Why do we now spend more than four times the 1971 amount ($2,500 adjusted for inflation) for health care per capita? It is too complicated to explain in a sentence, in a paragraph, or even over several pages. That's why I wrote this book.

In this book, I will discuss the means to solve the problems and reduce the high costs of health care. I will present the systems of health care used by other advanced countries in the world. The solutions are obvious. Just as no shoe fits all foot sizes, our country's solutions should be tailored to the strengths of our country. In the end, Congress holds the cards. All 535 senators and representatives must be bold enough to stand up to the health care industrial complex. Congress must refuse strings-attached political contributions and stop courting lobbyists from health plans, prescription drug corporations, health care hedge funds, hospitals, and others who place profit ahead of bedside care.

ONE

Prescription Drugs

Monopolies and Profits

KEY CONCEPTS

1. Big Pharma has created monopolies for many prescription drugs.
2. Congress has provided legal loopholes to allow these monopolies.
3. High prices have driven up costs for individuals and insurance companies.
4. Pharmaceutical corporations' lobbying and campaign donations influence Congress.

Pharmaceutical and health products money spent on lobbying in 2018: $281,000,000
Campaign contributions to congressional candidates in 2018: $29,076,000

If you are a student in one of my classes, you might think, "Prescription drugs. So what. I don't need any and never will." Wrong. Chances are your parents take one or more medications, and chances are even higher that your grandparents are on multiple prescription drugs. Put yourself in the shoes of your grandparents. They may be on a fixed monthly retirement of $1,200 from Social Security and, perhaps, a small pension; yet, they may face monthly prescription costs for medications of $500, $600, or even $1,000. High prescription drug prices have forced some Americans to travel to Mexico or Canada to buy prescription drugs at affordable prices.

When I went to medical school, most prescription drugs were cheap. Each step of the process—from chemical manufacture of a drug to distribution and retail sale—involved intense competition among drug manufacturers. Companies worried that if they set prices too high, someone would undercut them. Quality and service appeared to be an important element of the prescription drug sector.

Sadly, over the past half-century, high profits and Wall Street stock prices have become the driving force behind rising drug prices. Enter the monopoly model. Like many other sectors of the economy, large pharmaceutical companies—or Big Pharma—have placed a premium on massive profits, focusing on stock options, stock prices, and CEO compensation. Now the prescription medication business is targeted by Wall Street corporations, hedge funds, and private equity groups to take billions of dollars in excessive profits from the pockets of Americans using a set of tricks designed to fool all of us. Would you pay $50 for a $1 apple? Only if you were tricked. The trick in health care is to create a monopoly in the marketplace.

Some examples of high-priced drugs include the following:

1. Daraprim (generic) treats infections caused by microorganisms called protozoa: the cash price in 2014 was $13.50 a pill so that a 30-day supply cost $405. In 2015, the price was suddenly increased to $750 a pill, boosting the price for a 30-day supply to $22,500 just for profit.

2. Albendazole (generic) is prescribed for treatment of resistant pinworms in the United States and costs about two cents a pill to manufacture. It's sold wholesale to the World Health Organization for about two cents and used worldwide to treat many types of worms and intestinal parasitic infections. In the United States, albendazole sells in retail pharmacies for as much as $200 a pill. My office has received complaints from patients about this outrageous price, and albendazole costs were discussed in the prestigious *New England Journal of Medicine*.

3. Duexis is a prescription medication indicated to control pain and is usually prescribed for arthritis. It is a combination of two over-the-counter drugs, ibuprofen (Motrin), a common nonsteroidal anti-inflammatory drug (NSAID), and famotidine (Pepcid). Ibuprofen costs less than $10 for a bottle of 100 pills. Famotidine is added to reduce stomach acid and to decrease stomach inflammation, a side effect of ibuprofen. Famotidine sells for $20 for a bottle of 30 pills at a mom-and-pop drug store up the road from my office. When these two drugs are combined into one pill, the retail price (which includes a time-delay

agent) is about $3,000 for a month's supply. Later in this chapter, I will describe the hardship one of my patients faced after being prescribed a combination drug.

4. The EpiPen is an injectable device that administers epinephrine to treat a severe allergic reaction, or anaphylaxis. The price of a two-pack prescription suddenly jumped to $600 in 2016. Mylan, the company that markets EpiPen, had many excuses for the exorbitant price increase. An outraged public forced Congress to look into the matter. The company relented, a little, and offered a "discount" generic version, as well as discount coupons to those who figured out how to jump through the hoops. But the list price of the brand name purchased by schools, factories, municipalities, and other groups is still around $600. This made headlines during the 2016 election cycle (box 1.1).

The Legal Framework for Prescription Drugs and Medication

A complete discussion of all the federal laws and regulations that impact prescription drugs is beyond the scope of this book. Some with the greatest influence are discussed next.

US Patent Acts of 1790, 1836, 1861, 1952, and beyond. These acts provided exclusive markets for new inventions (and drugs), effectively giving the patent holder a monopoly of up to 20 years. This is the basis for the monopoly that companies have on new drugs that go to market. There is no price control on medications that are essential to life.

Pure Food and Drug Act of 1906. This law was in response to numerous deaths and illnesses from poisonous drugs. Before 1900, drugs and medicines were unregulated—a wild west of snake oil concoctions, pills, and syrups. President Teddy Roosevelt displayed true leadership for many laws that protected the public from bad food, bad drugs, and bad companies that took advantage of American workers.

The Pure Food and Drug Act of 1906 required that medications list the contents of all the ingredients on the label. The Bureau of Chemistry enforced labeling and tested the contents of medications to ensure that labels were truthful. In 1929, the Food and Drug Adminis-

Box 1.1

Many of my patients cannot afford their prescription drugs and never fill their prescriptions. While walking her dog one summer morning, one of my patients, Susan, was stung by a honeybee. Within a few moments, her skin blushed red, and she felt faint. A neighbor saw her slump to the sidewalk, and called 9-1-1. An ambulance arrived; the paramedics administered lifesaving epinephrine and transported her to a hospital emergency department. In the ED, she received additional treatments and was then discharged. The ED doctor cautioned her about bees and other stinging insects and advised her to wear an emergency bracelet. The doctor also wrote a prescription for an EpiPen, instructed her on how to use it, and warned her to carry it at all times.

She promptly went to one of several local pharmacies in the town where she lived. Shortly after handing her prescription to the pharmacist, she was told that her insurance company would not pay for the prescription. If she wanted the EpiPen Pak it would cost her nearly $600. She did not have the cash and had only a few dollars in her checking account. Her credit card debt was within a few dollars of her maximum limit. So she walked away without any epinephrine. At an office visit two weeks later, she asked me what she should do. I taught her how to use a small syringe and prescribed two vials of generic epinephrine, which she could afford.

That same summer, as a candidate for the US Congress, I produced a 60-second video describing the EpiPen as an example of Big Pharma gouging the public with outrageous prices. I told viewers how I place two vials of epinephrine in my first-aid kit, along with a small syringe. I order from a US distributor that sells to physicians, hospitals, and clinics. Each vial costs me $4 and contains enough epinephrine for three EpiPens.

And the epinephrine is made in the United States. It appears that too many drug companies use their corporate power to extort money from the good people in towns and cities across the United States. The EpiPen is the tip of the iceberg for unreasonable, greed-driven profit of so many pharmaceutical corporations.

tration (FDA) was created to police medication purity, taking over the job previously done by the Bureau of Chemistry.

Harrison Narcotic Act of 1914. This law was in response to numerous deaths from cocaine and narcotics. This act outlawed over-the-counter sale of narcotics and cocaine. These substances could only be obtained with a prescription written by a physician. Over the past 100 years, many updates have been enacted to regulate certain addicting prescription drugs; most important is the Controlled Substance Act of 1970.

Food, Drug, and Cosmetic Act of 1938. The event that stimulated passage of this law occurred when a new antibiotic sulfa drug was mixed with an elixir containing ethylene glycol, a toxic substance found in automobile radiator antifreeze, and administered orally to sick people. After numerous deaths, Congress passed this law, which mandated the safety of food and drugs and gave the FDA the authority to enforce the measure. The new, lengthy application process also required proof from the manufacturer of the medication's effectiveness.

Hatch-Waxman Act of 1986. This legislation was intended to make it easier for companies to introduce generic medications after a patent had expired. Before this act, if Company 1 had a patent on drug A that expired, and Company 2 wanted to make the same drug (drug A) as a generic, Company 2 would have had to navigate an impossible gauntlet of steps to get the generic approved. The Hatch-Waxman Act streamlined the process. But the law is filled with loopholes; therefore, it's easier for companies to gain monopolies on an array of drugs, ushering in look-alike drugs. Big Pharma lobbyists and campaign donations were no doubt behind many of the loopholes.

FDA regulatory actions (1986 to the present). Since 1986, the number of rules issued by the FDA has increased dramatically. Many of these new rules have benefited Big Pharma, not consumers. Members of Congress have arm-twisted the FDA to include regulations that benefit Big Pharma. If the FDA refuses to go along with requests by individual members of Congress, lawmakers can insert new rules into unrelated legislation. For example, a member of Congress can slip a loophole into a 1,000-page piece of legislation that is assured passage and certain to be signed into law. Does every member of Congress read all 1,000 pages of a proposed law? The answer is no, so the loophole goes unnoticed.

Medicare Prescription Drug, Improvement, and Modernization Act of 2003. The intent of the law was to help Medicare recipients pay for prescription drugs. However, it prevents Medicare from negotiating drug prices and has resulted in a huge windfall to pharmaceutical companies. One of my Medicare patients complained that a local pharmacy charged him $52 for one pill of Cialis. Cialis purchased in Europe in the generic form tadalafil costs less than $1 a pill, a price that includes drugstores' and the manufacturers' profits.

The Evolution of Prescription Drugs to a Monopoly Market

The business culture of free market capitalism began to shift in the 1980s from "profit is good" to "more profit is even better." This trend was noticed in the media and became the topic of several Hollywood films. In the 1987 film *Wall Street*, superstar Michael Douglas is depicted as the fictional character Gordon Gekko whose motto is "greed is good." Some in the prescription drug business seem to have taken up this motto.

Big Pharma has developed and refined a series of methods over the past 30 years designed to maximize profits. One of the most successful marketing methods is to create an exclusive monopoly on a drug and set the price high enough to make an outrageous profit. American corporations' first priority is to make a profit benefiting stockholders in the form of dividends and increased stock prices. It follows that large bonuses to corporate officers and CEOs are expected. Moral and social norms have been thrown aside, and the US Congress has removed many of the detours and roadblocks to price gouging.

Outrageous prices for many prescription drugs and over-the-counter medications have driven up the cost of health care for millions of people. A new monopoly opportunity has been created with the development of a class of drugs commonly referred to as biologics. Most biologics target certain types of immune system cells that modulate our immune system. Imagine a vast array of hundreds of circuit breakers in a 20-story office building. By switching off the correct circuit breaker, you could stop the annoying elevator music. In the human body, an antibody can be injected that can turn off any one of hundreds of immune functions. In the case of rheumatoid arthritis, an antibody can be manufactured that stops an immune attack on human joints that causes arthritis and pain. Such antibodies can be mass-produced with ease in the laboratory using recombinant DNA technology.

The poster child for monoclonal drugs is adalimumab (Humira). This agent is used in the treatment of rheumatoid arthritis. It is a new class of agents advertised on TV to reduce pain and stop further joint damage. These are monoclonal antibodies, mass-produced in commercial laboratories that alter our immune and inflammatory systems. What the TV ad does not provide us is the sticker price for Humira: it costs in the range of $5,000 a month, or $60,000 for a year of treatment. And these new biologics are the darlings of Wall Street, targeting conditions that include multiple sclerosis, ulcerative colitis, psoriasis, some cancers, and many other conditions. Some come at a price tag of over $200,000 a year. The FDA has proposed listing of wholesale prices on TV ads, but the proposal is strongly opposed by the pharmaceutical lobby.

Rebranding Generics to Gain a Monopoly

At the beginning of this chapter, I listed a few examples of common everyday prescription drugs that I use in my clinical practice that have outrageous prices. Some, like the insulins, are basically generic. The patent rights to insulin were given to the University of Toronto in 1923 by scientists who stipulated that anyone could produce it without paying royalties. A month's supply of insulin pens can now cost $500. A month's supply of insulin should cost $30 to $50. As of 2019, Walmart Pharmacy still sold old formulations of insulin for $30, enough for several weeks, depending on the daily dose needed.

Through a variety of tricks, pharmaceutical companies have created "patents" by making minor tweaks to drugs. They have created monopolies for many drugs, either by buying out the competition or by fine-tuning the drug to be slightly molecularly different but clinically the same. Another trick is "secret collusion": raise the price of a drug and expect the competition will do the same. Open collusion is illegal, but what if two CEOs of competing drug companies have a short conversation on the golf course?

In addition to the examples of high-priced prescription drugs I listed at the beginning of the chapter, listed below are more examples of price gouging:

Insulin. Numerous forms of insulin are available, including dial-a-dose insulin pens. The insulin pen improves safety but at a cost of $400 to $500 for a month's supply. Contrast this to common prices of $10 to $20 for insulin not so long ago.

Doxycycline. I commonly prescribe doxycycline, an oral antibiotic, in my practice. It is effective for bronchitis, pneumonia, sinusitis, otitis, and many other infections. Doxycycline can also be taken to prevent malaria. This generic drug has been used clinically since I was in medical school in the 1970s. A typical prescription consists of 20 tablets taken two a day for 10 days. Cost now ranges from $30 to $90. In 2011, 20 tablets cost only $5. The news media have reported on this price increase and blamed it on quality control. I believe it also increased profits.

Acetazolamide and its cousins. Some old drugs now have new prices. I like adventure travel to far corners of the earth, places both remote and hard to get to. I have trekked in Nepal to elevations of 18,000 feet above sea level, where the atmospheric pressure is half that of sea level, and, hence, the amount of oxygen with each inhaled breath is also half. To prevent altitude sickness, most people trekking to these high elevations take medication. Most popular is acetazolamide (Diamox), which is also used by eye specialists to treat glaucoma. When I first ventured to high elevations, acetazolamide cost five cents a pill, which was still the cost in Kathmandu in 2018. But if you pick it up beforehand in the United States, it's a dollar a pill—20 times higher than what it should cost. That's a lot of profit.

Another example is the brother of acetazolamide, a generic medication called diclofenamide (Daranide). It's similar to acetazolamide because it inhibits an enzyme that is important in CO_2 transport and is classified as a carbonic anhydrase inhibitor.

This old glaucoma drug was reborn as an orphan drug for a disease called periodic paralysis. Patients with periodic paralysis can wake up paralyzed. They may go through their days feeling as if they are wearing lead shoes and a 40-pound lead trench coat. Its list price was $50 a bottle in 2002. Congress passed a law to reclassify it as an orphan drug. Strongbridge Biopharma relaunched it, with a new brand name—Keveyis—and a new price: $15,000 a bottle. That's over $180,000 a year for treatment. Credit Suisse analysts estimated the drug could bring in $100 million per year for Taro Pharma.

An orphan drug is used to treat rare diseases and hence has limited sales. The trick used to create Keveyis is the special protection granted by Congress under the Orphan Drug Act of 1983. Intended to promote marketing of medications for rare diseases, industry looked at this as an opportunity to gain monopoly status on the marketplace. So if you desperately need an orphan drug, Big Pharma can charge any amount they like. No price regulation. And they know they can force insurance companies to pay $1,000 for a 10-cent pill.

Mom-and-Pop Small Pharmacies Are Being Replaced with Corporate Pharmacies

When I first began my career as a doctor, most of the pharmacies where patients obtained their prescription drugs were small single owner businesses. As a practicing physician, I can tell you I would prefer to interact with a small pharmacy where I could get to know the first names of staff, who were generally happy, patient, and friendly, and could solve problems and prescription misunderstandings and errors quickly. If one pharmacy did not provide good service, there were many others to choose from. I find talking to most corporate pharmacy staff less appealing for many reasons; first I have to navigate a complex maze of an impersonal phone tree, then talk with detached staff, only to be placed on hold, and finally speak with a hurried pharmacist. Finally, add the new requirement for electronic prescriptions and things get even worse. I now have to search through a list of diagnoses and add that to the electronic prescription. That takes extra time. Sometimes the prescription never arrives at the pharmacy, to the distress of the patient. And now certain health plans only allow prescriptions to be filled at their preferred corporate pharmacy, unless the patient wants to pay full price. The 2018 merger between Aetna and CVS exemplifies the close association among health plans and pharmacies.

Tricks to Keep the Monopoly Business Model in Place

Pharmaceutical companies use many methods to extract profits from prescription drugs; some legal, some deceitful.

Trick 1: Combine cheap drugs to make an expensive one. I talked about Duexis in the introduction to this chapter. There are many others. In my medical practice, I cared for a delightful, energetic 80-year-old woman for many years. Sadly, she had a stroke that left her partially paralyzed, and she worked hard to regain full activities. The hospitalist (see chapter 3, "Physicians") sent her home with a prescription for Aggrenox, which is a combination of two drugs: aspirin and dipyridamole. The hospital pharmacy charged her nearly $500. She did not have Medicare Part D, so she put the cost on her charge card. When I saw her, she wanted a refill prescription for Aggrenox, but that stretched her budget. I had a solution. Take one aspirin a day (which costs pennies) plus a generic dipyridamole, which costs $60 for a month's supply. She and her partner were shocked. Why did the hospital send them home with a $500 prescription when $60 plus an aspirin would have done the trick?

Trick 2: Fool the doctors. Persuading doctors to prescribe new brand name prescription drugs is a big business, as described in trick 1. How is this done? By persuading doctors to prescribe the drug that makes the most profit for pharmaceutical companies. Big Pharma employs armies of salespersons to persuade doctors to prescribe their drug. Pfizer employs upward of 10,000 people in its sales force. (The movie *Love & Other Drugs*, starring Anne Hathaway, offers entertaining insight into the world of pharmaceutical sales forces.)

Why do so many physicians prescribe superexpensive drugs to their patients? In many cases, the physicians don't have a clue as to the list price of the drug. I have had contact with many pharmaceutical sales-people during my career—in the office, at university-level continuing medical education conferences, and at an "educational dinner" orga-nized by a pharmaceutical corporation. If I ask, "How much does drug XYZ cost?" the reflex answer is, "It's covered by most insurance." When I probe deeper, requesting they disclose the actual list price, I never get a straight answer. They squirm, and respond, "There are spe-cial programs for patients who cannot afford it." If I really want to know the price of a drug, I have to call the pharmacy.

The pharmaceutical sales representatives, also known as the *drug detail person*, often provide physicians with beautifully illustrated glossy handouts on the benefits of the drug they promote. Usually, they will distribute copies of medical journal articles that support use of their drug. Most doctors are too busy to read these journal articles be-yond the abstract. They miss the fact that, too often, some authors received funding from Big Pharma or that the drug is only minimally effective. They take the word of the pharmaceutical representative.

Thirty years ago, pharmaceutical companies courted doctors with free baseball tickets, ski lift tickets, hotel rooms, dinners, clothing, pens, paper, and more. I was once given a nice baseball cap by a drug rep-resentative (rep), which displayed the name of a new drug. When the drug was recalled, the rep wanted the cap returned to him. (I had a Viagra tie, given to me as a gift from Pharma, but my wife made me throw it away.) Fortunately, most of these subconscious bribes have been prohibited by rules adapted by the Pharmaceutical Research and Manufactures of America (PhRMA) a major pharmaceutical trade organization after pressure from consumer groups.

Trick 3: Hold health plans hostage. Why aren't more people scream-ing their heads off over these outrageous drug prices? Because many people are lucky; they may only have to pay a small co-pay of $10 or $20. Their insurance has to cover the rest of the cost.

Jill, a friend of mine, has multiple sclerosis (MS) and takes a medi-cation called teriflunomide (Aubagio) that has slowed progression of her disease. She is grateful that the medication has helped her, and that she is still able to hike on mountain trails. This drug sells retail for

$8,000 for a month's supply, a price so prohibitive that only the very wealthy can pay out of pocket. However, a health plan could pay. Initially, many health plans refused to pay, but then the MS support groups and physicians began to scream that not paying for drugs will cause people to die. This in effect holds the health plan hostage.

When health care insurance companies pay for outrageous drug costs, these costs are ultimately passed on to consumers and employers in the form of higher premiums.

Trick 4: Eliminate the competition. Here is a case from my days of working in emergency departments (EDs). A young woman arrived in the ED by ambulance. She was psychotic, or what we call agitated delirium. She was screaming, yelling, arching her back, and flailing her arms about in the air. The paramedics restrained her with cloth straps to prevent the woman from hurting herself and others. She admitted to using methamphetamine, and the paramedics confirmed that others in the house where they picked her up said she "took too much speed."

I turned to the nurse in the resuscitation room and said, "Get me 10 milligrams (mg) of IV droperidol, stat."

"We don't have it in the Pyxis [a locked machine that stores drugs] anymore," she replied. "They finally took it away from us."

I knew of attempts to take away this lifesaving drug from the hands of ED doctors but did not know it would happen so soon. I ordered a different IV drug to help stop her agitated delirium and prevent its complications. Why didn't we use diazepam (Valium) in the first place? Because my colleagues and I had published several scientific research studies that showed that droperidol worked best as an antidote to methamphetamine agitation.

How could an essential drug be taken away from American EDs? My colleagues in the ED began to investigate, and even published a scholarly article after surveying many other EDs. We found that a handful of unsubstantiated reports led the FDA to place a black box warning on the drug. We suspected that the manufacturer of a new brand name drug may have had something to do with the reports sent to the FDA, but could not prove it. And that new drug did not work as well for agitated ED patients.

Trick 5: Promote dangerous drugs to make a profit. Drugs that can harm people can also raise a drug corporation's stock price. Rofecoxib, a COX-2 inhibitor, is a pain medication in a class of drugs called NSAIDs. It was marketed under the brand name Vioxx beginning in 1999 and prescribed to millions of people. It was patent protected, so the company has a monopoly on the drug and used its clout to heavily market to doctors. Touted as a miracle drug, it contributed to the rise in Merck's stock price, but it also caused increased heart attacks, strokes, and other problems. Vioxx was finally pulled from the market, and Merck agreed to a mass tort settlement of $4.8 billion. Court proceedings showed that the corporation had withheld data showing the dangers of Vioxx.

Trick 6: Exaggerate cures on media, especially TV. Amid the 2017–18 flu season, I examined a 50-year-old woman with a severe case of influenza. She had a fever, weakness, profound fatigue, muscle aches, sore throat, and a horrible cough for about a week. The rapid flu test we did in the office tested positive for influenza A. She asked for a prescription for oseltamivir (Tamiflu), because the TV ads had led her to believe it would cure her. I explained that it would have no benefit if started beyond 48 hours of symptom onset. Scientific literature indicated that the most benefit occurred if the drug was started within 28 hours of the onset of symptoms. Even if started early, the benefit is limited: it can reduce illness from seven to six days. "But the TV ad says it will cure me," she argued.

Oseltamivir had been promoted worldwide as a treatment for influenza A. Hoffman-La Roche, the multinational, multibillion-dollar company that sells oseltamivir, has patent protection. A prescription for the standard seven-day course—two pills a day (75 mg) costs nearly $100. As a professor at the University of California, Davis, I lecture on influenza, and have done so for the past 25 years. So I know the inside story and much of the published scientific research on influenza. When oseltamivir was first introduced, I was invited and paid by Hoffman-La Roche to give a lecture on influenza to a group of practicing physicians. I was never invited to give a second lecture by the corporation, I think because

I told the truth, that the drug only reduced symptoms by a day. Of course, every few months or so, I update my PowerPoint lecture, as volumes of medical studies continue to pour into the scientific literature. During flu season, at least one patient a day tells me about this "great medication" advertised on TV and asks if I can write them a prescription.

Direct-to-consumer advertising for a wide range of prescription drugs is rampant. During prime-time programming chances are you will see a 30-second ad telling you about a wonder cure and to "talk to your doctor." Direct-to-consumer advertising occurs through TV, radio, magazine, the internet, and other media. My patients, who come to me requesting a miracle drug for a variety of medical problems, are disappointed when I discuss the facts of the advertised drug. Often our conversation goes like this: "It will not work for your condition. There are better drugs that have fewer serious side effects. Do you want to pay $50 a month for 95% relief or $6,000 a month for 96% relief? Oh, and by the way, the expensive drug has many more side effects; some that can harm you."

Physician and consumer groups have called for an end to direct-to-consumer advertising of prescription drugs, but Congress ignores these pleas. Perhaps because of the millions of dollars that Big Pharma contributes to their election campaigns. The TV ads continue, with hundreds of colorful ads, happy people, and nice music. I recently counted over 10 different Humira ads with these happy people who tell you about the alleged benefits of the drug in relieving their arthritis pain.

Does the reader remember the last lines in TV ads? Most often they say, "Talk to your doctor about taking drug X-Y-Z." I would therefore expect hundreds of scientists to be knocking on my office door eager to explain the side effects and harm that can be inflicted by the advertised drug. I am still waiting. Instead, an occasional pharmaceutical representative would come to the office to explain the benefits of a drug they are selling and hand me a colorful brochure: the side effects listed in print so small I need a magnifying glass to read it.

Trick 7: Cheating and fraud. The US Office of Inspector General (OIG) has authority, like a cop on the beat, to catch pharmaceutical companies that cheat or engage in fraudulent activity. A recent example includes a $785 million settlement made to the US Department of Justice with Pfizer and Wyeth to settle *allegations* of fraud. The settlement was made to resolve allegations that Wyeth knowingly reported to the government false and fraudulent prices on two of its proton pump inhibitor (PPI) drugs, Protonix Oral and Protonix IV. Pfizer acquired Wyeth in 2009.

Trick 8: Price fixing of generics. Price fixing occurs when companies collude to set prices, thus eliminating free market competition and creating a monopoly. On December 9, 2018, the *Washington Post* published an article on price fixing of generic drugs, involving 300 different prescription drugs. In one case, albuterol, a generic asthma medication, had its price raised 3,400%.

The US Senate Investigates the Monopoly Business Model

In 2016, the US Senate got wind of the outrageous increases in prescription drug prices and convened a focused investigation. Senator Susan Collins (R-ME) chaired the Special Committee on Aging that published its report in December 2016 titled *Sudden Price Spikes in Off-Patent Prescription Drugs: The Monopoly Business Model That Harms Patients, Taxpayers, and the U.S. Health Care System* (S. Rep. No. 114-429 [2015–16]).

The report focused on four investor-backed pharmaceutical companies that developed business models designed to eliminate any free market competition and create a monopoly for certain drugs. This monopoly allowed these companies to raise prices as much as 5,000%; therefore, a $20 drug could be increased to $1,000. Who can afford that and still put food on the table?

An excerpt from the US Senate report describes the devastating impact on people:

> In May 2015, when Isla Weston was just two months old, doctors diagnosed her with a life-threatening parasitic infection known as toxoplasmosis. Immediate treatment was needed to cure this infection;

otherwise, the parasite would attack vital cells in the little girl's brain, potentially leaving her with lifelong deficits in cognition and function—or even causing her death.

Isla was prescribed Daraprim, the standard of care, which would cure the active infection in a year. To the shock and dismay of the infant's family, and other Americans who relied on this vital medicine, the price of the 63-year-old drug that this child desperately needed had just spiked from $13.50 a tablet to $750 a tablet, an increase of more than 5,000 percent, in just one day.

Testifying at a 2016 Senate Special Committee on Aging hearing, held just a few days after Isla's first birthday, her mother, Shannon Weston, described the impact of that staggering price tag:

> I was hopeless and depressed at the thought of what would happen to my perfect little girl if I was not able to help her. . . . I looked into any way I could think of to come up with the almost $360,000 necessary to treat my daughter for a year with a drug that she needed, knowing that as long as she was treated before symptoms set in she would remain asymptomatic.

How many of us have $360,000 tucked under our mattress ready to hand over to an investor-owned entity to pay for pills that actually cost less that $1 to produce? The four companies investigated by the US Senate included Turing, Retrophin, Rodelis, and Valeant. Examples of generic drugs, listed here by their brand name, that they used to gain monopoly control of prices follow:

> Seromycin: $500 for a 30-day supply, increased to $10,800
> Cuprimine: $445 for a 30-day supply, increased to $35,000
> Daraprim: $405 for a 30-day supply, increased to $22,500
> Isuprel: $218 for a single-dose vial, increased to $1,790

The result of the Senate investigation? No legislation was immediately passed into law to stop price gouging because of pharmaceutical lobbying efforts and campaign donations to Congress.

Steps to Stop Outrageous Prescription Prices

Most developed countries—including those with very conservative governments—have employed effective solutions to control drug costs, which is why people in these countries often pay less than half of what people in the United States pay for drugs. Congress can control the purse strings of drug prices. Congress must act with tough, straightforward solutions, not with thousands of pages of loopholes. We the people must also make noise to get Congress to pass legislation that benefits bedside medicine, not corporate medicine. People can do this both as an individual with letters, e-mails, and calls to members of Congress and as members of advocacy groups. And don't forget to vote.

I have listed below a number of steps that should be taken to reduce the price of prescription drugs. These include:

1. *Federal campaign finance reform: Prohibit political campaign contributions to members of Congress by Big Pharma.* How can a US senator or representative vote in the best interest of the people when large campaign contributions come from corporations? Getting reelected costs millions of dollars, and a history of voting in favor of corporations increases the likelihood of receiving more corporate donations. Examples of money donated to campaign committees of members of Congress in the 2018 election cycle by Pharmaceuticals/Health Products listed by OpenSecrets include

Sen. Bob Casey (D): $538,000
Rep. Greg Walden (R): $458,000
Sen. John Barrasso (R): $229,000
Rep. Frank Pallone (D): $247,000

Will legislators ever vote to put the brakes on outrageous drug prices?

2. *Prohibit lobbying by the pharmaceutical industry.* Big Pharma is well represented on Capitol Hill with an army of lobbyists. They meet with our representatives and senators with a long list of one-sided reasons to enact laws that benefit pharmaceutical companies at

the expense of the American people. As noted at the beginning of this chapter, nearly $300 million was spent by pharma/health products in 2018 lobbying Congress. Lobbyists often get their foot in the door with big smiles, the unspoken prospect of a future campaign contribution.

3. *Enforce and strengthen anti-monopoly laws.* This country was built on free enterprise, but a monopoly on any product or any drug allows the manufacturer/distributor to charge any price and set astronomically high prices. The public must choose between paying exorbitant prices or facing financial ruin or even death. Monopolies have been around a long time, and history has shown that only government has been successful in trust busting. Corporations should be prohibited from controlling multiple drug companies that make generics and set outrageous prices. Currently, many drugs are manufactured overseas but imported by US companies that jack up the price. Why does a drug made in India then imported to the United States cost $50 a pill but $2 a pill in Europe?

4. *Prohibit proprietary patents on combination pills.* A common practice is to paste two inexpensive generic drugs together in the same single pill and then claim patent protection. As a physician, I hate this. How do I adjust a dose when a patient with hypertension is on 20 mg of lisinopril and 25 mg of hydrochlorothiazide (HCTZ) if I only want to increase the lisinopril to 30 mg and leave the HCTZ dose the same? An example of a rip-off price is Prempro (for meno-pausal symptoms). This drug's retail price can be as much as $195 for a 30-day supply. It is a combination of estrogens and medroxyproges-terone, each of which can be purchased separately for less than $15.

5. *Reduce patent protection time for new drugs.* Corporations claim they need extensive patent times to recover research costs. Much of the basic drug research is done in universities that use taxpayer-funded grants from the National Institutes of Health. Shortening patent protection of new drugs would lower prices and decrease out-of-pocket expenses. Yes, it costs money to bring a new drug to market through phase 1, 2, and 3 studies. But should com-panies reap billions of dollars in profit?

6. *Outlaw new patents on look-a-like drugs.* When a new drug nears the end of patent protection, a tiny tweak can be made to the chemical structure to qualify it as a new drug, even though it has the same clinical effect. A corporation gets additional years of exclusive patent protection and the accompanying high price tag. Big Pharma can block potential competition from companies wanting to make the old generic drug through loopholes in the law.

7. *Adapt a European model: Require competitive negotiation for government programs.* Prices for prescription drugs should be negotiated similar to advanced European countries. The negotiating table should include physicians, politicians, patients, health plans, hospitals, and the prescription drug industry. Start with prescription drugs paid through federal programs, including Medicare, Medicaid, Veterans Affairs, the military, and TRICARE. Then expand price negotiation to include all health plans and cash-paying patients. To this end, Speaker of the House Nancy Pelosi introduced the Elijah E. Cummings Lower Drug Costs Now Act (H.R. 3) on September 19, 2019.

8. *Require cost-benefit analysis of certain drugs.* A cost-benefit analysis should be performed before any federal money can be spent on drugs. Poorly effective drugs would not be approved for federal programs. For example, Opdivo is an anticancer drug that costs $150,000—for an extra three months of life, while attached to an oxygen tube and miserable.

Bottom line: The excessive influence of Big Pharma on the US Congress needs to be curtailed. Through legislative loopholes, Big Pharma has been gifted monopolies that result in outrageous prescription drug prices.

TWO

Hospitals

Profit First

KEY CONCEPTS

1. Over the past 30 years, single hospitals have consolidated into large chains, creating monopolies that drive up health care costs.
2. Hospital prices may be double or triple actual costs and what Medicare pays.
3. Half of this increase results from improved technology and advances in medical care. But the other 50% is unnecessary and results from excessive profits, executive compensation, administrative inefficiency, and burdensome operational rules and regulations.
4. In the era of bedside medicine, hospitals served doctors; now doctors serve hospitals.
5. Patient care protocols can result in unnecessary testing and procedures and increased hospital profits.

Hospital and nursing home money spent on lobbying in 2018: $100,962,000
Campaign contributions to congressional candidates in 2018: $17,972,000

Our education system, from kindergarten to high school, teaches us that hospitals are good: They cure the sick and heal the injured. They can do miraculous things like transplant hearts and replace broken and worn-out joints. Many Americans think highly of hospitals, even donating hard-earned dollars to annual fund drives. But now hospitals operate on a Wall Street business model and inflate retail prices for their services to 2, 3, or even 10 times the actual cost. Their billing and collection services are not your warm, fuzzy friends: they harass, threaten, and intimidate patients and will send unpaid accounts to ruthless collection agencies. "America's Hospitals Are a Racket," proclaimed the *Economist*, a respected international news journal, in the November 23, 2019, issue. Does anyone ever end up bankrupt and

One of my patients came to the office for an adjustment of heart medications. I noticed dried blood on the scrapped knuckles of his hands.

"What happened?" I asked.

"I pull the rotor out of my distributer cap every night so I don't get my pickup truck stolen, I mean repossessed. I scraped my hands last night," he said. "I worry about debt collectors stealing my only possession, my old rusty pickup truck. I live in a mobile home park, so I don't have a garage. The hospital says I owe them $120,000, but that's a lie."

Randy had developed breathing trouble when he was 200 miles from home in the central valley of California. The 55-year-old unemployed mechanic went to a hospital emergency department, where he was diagnosed with a pulmonary embolism (blood clot to the lungs) and was hospitalized for five days. His course was complicated by an underlying condition of congestive heart failure. At discharge, the hospital refused to give him a $600 prescription for a blood thinning medication because he had no money or credit card. Now he received harassing phone calls from the hospital's finance department. They threatened to send him to a collection agency.

Yet he is on California's Medicaid program, which prohibits hospitals from going after patients to pay for their bills. Hospitals must accept what Medicaid pays and not balance bill the patient. But his Medicaid had expired, and he told me his application to be placed back on the program was lost in bureaucracy. The hospital did not care. They just wanted their money. Randy said the hospital was in the process of turning over his debt to a collection agency. As we will discuss later in this chapter, hospitals sell debt for pennies on the dollar to collection agencies.

homeless as a result of hospital bills? Yes. It happens all the time, including to some of my patients (box 2.1).

Hospital Charges and Fees

Hospitals employ many people; the largest hospitals employ thousands of people. Hospital care costs money and directly or indirectly someone has to pay for salaries, supplies, and building costs. Examples of charges from bills I have reviewed:

1. Hip replacement (3 days): $102,000
2. Emergency department (ED) evaluation of abdominal pain (9 hours): $21,000
3. Intensive care unit (ICU) admission for pneumonia (5 days): $246,000

How are these prices determined? Many charges are arbitrary, randomly determined by a bean counter without any real knowledge of the frontline delivery of care. It is not unusual for prices to be two or three times the actual cost of care.

Over time, hospitals throughout America have justified rebranding themselves as medical centers that provide more than EDs and acute inpatient beds. Hospitals have added outpatient services and fee-for-service charges too. The focus is now on profit and revenue. Millionaire CEOs and administrators compete for huge annual bonuses based less on good patient care and more on revenue streams. Before we discuss corporate prices, rules, and structure, let's review the different types of hospitals and their evolution from village friendliness to impersonal profit centers.

Hospital Structure

For the purpose of this chapter, medical centers and hospitals will be collectively referred to as hospitals. Nearly 7,000 hospitals existed in 1975. The number of hospitals has declined over the past 40 years. Currently, nearly 5,000 acute care hospitals exist in the United States. Up until the 1960s, most hospitals were locally owned and controlled. Thirty years ago, hospitals served physicians, who in turn served ill and injured patients. Too often now, the hospital serves a corporate culture that follows a Wall Street script, richly rewarding senior executives.

I have watched the personal touch of caring and helping people fade away. In its place are impersonal hospital rules designed to enhance profit. But these regulations are often justified for patient safety and regulatory compliance.

Hospitals fall into one of several categories, including community, district, teaching, county government, and federal facilities.

Community Hospitals

Community hospitals comprise the vast majority of hospitals and can be sorted into for-profit and not-for-profit. They can be further subdivided as religion-based and non-religion-based hospitals. Non-religion-based hospitals are owned and operated by private groups or companies and can be either for-profit or nonprofit. They make money by charging patients fees in order to operate. Over the past 30 years, smaller freestanding hospitals have been bought by larger hospitals, forming hospital systems, or hospital chains. As of 2019, examples of for-profit systems include Hospital Corporation of America (HCA) with more than 180 hospitals, Community Health Systems with more than 100 hospitals, and Tenet with more than 60 hospitals. The entities that create hospital systems include private equity groups, Wall Street corporations, nonprofit enterprises, and others. Common reasons put forth for consolidating hospitals include economies of scale, improved service to patients, and new efficiencies. But some economists argue that buying independent small- and medium-sized hospitals creates a monopoly. When all hospitals in a region have the same owner, higher prices can be charged resulting in higher profits.

Some small hospitals have closed or have been merged into large hospital systems because of their inability to purchase expensive technology, meet big city standards of medical care, or comply with overburdensome regulations. Still others have faced financial problems because a disproportionate number of patients are uninsured. Consolidated hospitals create monopolies, charge higher prices, and hold patients and insurers hostage. A recent study showed that large systems provide worse care than single hospitals. In addition, impersonal service, billing errors, and the practice of medicine by corporate protocols, make consolidation bad for the average person.

The majority of acute care hospitals are chartered as nonprofit businesses. One might think that nonprofit hospitals are warm and fuzzy places that put the public good first. They are required by law to provide a community benefit, and many have spent money on projects that truly benefit the community. However, some have earmarked community benefit funds to offset losses from low-paying Medicaid rates and media reports have cautioned that community benefits may be less than assumed. Many of these hospitals operate on a corporate model and jump through a few governmental regulatory hoops to qualify as nonprofit, meaning they pay no federal income taxes. Many of these CEOs collect more than $1 million a year in salary and bonuses, and top hospital executives can make nearly that much. How do they hide their profits? Enormous profits can be hidden by paying large bonuses to senior executives, hiding money in reserves, donating to other organizations, earmarking money for nonexistent future projects, spending money on inefficient administrative projects, and other means.

Religion-based hospitals, also referred to as faith-based hospitals, are owned and operated by religious organizations, and most are chartered as nonprofits. These include Catholic, Baptist, Adventist, Methodist, and other hospitals. Many began as individual freestanding hospitals but over the past 30 years have linked together or consolidated to form hospital systems across wide areas of America. In the past, they provided discounted or free care, making up losses with donations from the parent religious organization. But in growing large, they have adapted a corporate model of business, with associated high retail prices. Recently, Dignity Health, formerly Mercy Hospital Systems (36 hospitals), merged with Catholic Health Initiatives to form Common Spirit Health, comprising 142 hospitals in a $29 billion system. Adventist Health operates 45 hospitals, and Trinity Health Systems 92 hospitals. I recently had a simple x-ray taken of my right foot at an Adventist hospital. The retail charge listed was nearly $500 for an $80 x-ray according to Medicare rules.

District Hospitals

Local government hospital boards own and operate district hospitals. District hospitals are chartered to provide citizen-community governance of services. Boundaries may include a small area of a county, an entire county, or parts of several counties. Voters elect hospital governing boards in regular elections to oversee the operation. The voters within the district in theory decide the makeup of the governing board and can remove ineffective members through recall. These hospitals use a combination of funds collected from patients, taxpayer revenue, and funding drives. Many communities are proud of their district hospital and participate in fundraising.

Fewer district hospitals exist now compared to 30 years ago for several reasons: (1) federal and state regulations are beyond their financial means, (2) flight of specialists to metropolitan areas, (3) expense of high technology such as MRIs, and (4) and acquisition by national mega-hospital groups.

Teaching Hospitals

Teaching hospitals, often referred to as Academic Medical Centers, are usually owned or affiliated with medical schools and universities and focus on teaching, research, and patient care. Nearly all of the main campus hospitals are nonprofit. While they charge patients for care, they also collect revenue through grants and government subsidies. Paradoxically, their prices for care are now among the highest of all hospitals, even though they use discount labor: interns and residents provide the bulk of physician patient care. Children's hospitals provide specialized care only for children and are most often teaching hospitals. Academic Medical Centers can expand their reach by merging and acquiring other hospitals, forming large systems. Several examples stand out. The Yale New Haven Health system created a virtual monopoly by purchasing several hospitals in Connecticut. The West Virginia University Health System purchased several hospitals in West Virginia, even closing one, St. Joseph's in Parkersburg, West Virginia, thus creating a monopoly-like environment and higher prices. Over 50% of the hospital beds in Pittsburgh, Pennsylvania, are operated by the University of Pittsburgh Medical Center system which has been accused of charging high prices.

HMO Hospitals

Health maintenance organizations may combine services of a health insurance plan, clinics, and hospitals as a single entity, all under one roof so to speak. This is discussed in more detail in chapter 4 on "Health Plans." The best known in this HMO group is the Kaiser Permanente Healthcare System. Kaiser operates community hospitals some of which also serve as teaching hospitals. Most of my patients have only good things to say about Kaiser, and my interaction with Kaiser physicians has been excellent. The Kaiser System appears to me to be a cost-efficient and quality-driven means of delivering health care.

Government Hospitals

Among government hospitals are Veterans Affairs hospitals, military hospitals, and local county hospitals. County hospitals are owned by county governments, initially created to care for patients with no or limited funding. Revenue from county governments is sometimes used to make up operating losses. In the past, physicians had a major voice in setting policy by serving on governing bodies. The physician governing body also oversaw the hospital director and nursing directors and could hire and fire. Now, administrators have more power and set many rules and regulations that physicians must follow. County hospitals are frequently affiliated with medical schools and rely on interns and residents to provide medical care. Some hospitals use a corporate model of charging high prices, and patients may receive a Ritz-Carlton bill for a Motel 6 bed.

Cancer Centers

Many cancer centers are divisions or sections of a hospital, although they may be located in separate geographical localities. Others are owned and operated by private corporations. Cancer centers provide diagnostic tests, studies, and treatments, such as certain IV chemotherapy infusions, which traditionally were performed in hospitals. Cancer centers are discussed in this chapter because of their corporate structure, high prices, and large profits.

Why Are Hospital Retail Fees So High?

There are both legitimate as well as inappropriate reasons for the evolution of hospitals into systems that have raised prices to unimaginable levels. Some drivers of increased fees are legitimate.

Well-intentioned government regulations can result in micromanaging hospital operations with redundant, overbearing, costly, and sometimes unnecessary rules. Some regulations are hundreds of pages long. Examples include remodel and new construction requirements, micromanagement of hospital staffing, redundant requirements for review of patient care, excessive demands for physician staff privileges, and requirements for data collection and input data. For example, California earthquake standards make new construction prohibitively expensive.

In addition, government regulations result in hiring extra staff, providing extra training, and requiring additional testing of patients, as well as time-consuming reporting requirements. Hospitals hire people to ensure compliance with rules. Nongovernment agencies also set rules and standards if a hospital wants to receive a specialty certification or accreditation. To be a certified trauma center, a hospital must comply with rules set by the American College of Surgeons.

The increase in complexity in the delivery of hospital care has also increased the cost of business. Medical care has evolved and improved over the past 30 years. Patients have benefited from new diagnostic techniques, cancer treatments, and new complex surgical techniques.

ICUs. Specialized units began to pop up in hospitals in the 1960s. ICUs aimed to care for critically ill people needing labor intensive care. Cardiac care units with newly adapted cardiac monitoring and medications decreased deaths from heart attacks. Surgical ICUs, neonatal ICUs, and pediatric ICUs improved the care of patients.

EDs. When I first began working in EDs, the goal of the physician was to decide who was sick or non-sick. Sick patients got admitted, and the admitting physician could figure out the cause. Non-sick included minor injuries, lacerations, fractures, and burns which we quickly cared for and sent home. Now EDs have evolved to one-stop shopping, where dozens of lab tests may be done with rapid results, and imaging that goes well beyond the x-ray, and includes CT scans, MRIs, and ultrasound. Newer tests are expensive, driving up costs, and slowing down EDs' patient flow.

Imaging. Advanced technology, including CT scans, MRIs, electron beam devices, ultrasound, and others, increase hospital costs. I have witnessed the impressive improvement in the standard of care as a result of these studies.

Specialty procedures. Surgical specialties have advanced technical procedures that may involve special instruments (i.e., tools) that improve patient outcomes but are very expensive for the hospital to purchase. Examples include vascular surgery; cardiac surgery; urology; neurosurgery; obstetrics-gynecology; ear, nose, throat; and many others, including the dreaded colonoscopy. Finally, submitting bills for payment to health insurance plans, and fighting the gauntlet of rules and refusals, can require an expensive army of workers.

Price Gouging

Advances in medical care might justify about half of the increases in hospital charges that have occurred since the 1980s. That just brings us to the current European costs of hospital care. The other half of the increased costs in American hospital can mostly be attributed to factors like inefficient management, wasting money on unneeded projects, high administrative salaries, and excessive profits on the many services they provide. In my opinion, this is wrong. These increases are inappropriate and derived from the monopoly business model of extreme profits.

Profit increases with increasing prices. Hospitals can arbitrarily set high prices, and there is nothing to stop them. Unlike buying most goods and services in a free market economy, hospitals do not advertise their prices. Some retail prices might be posted online but are often difficult to find. Who has time to shop around in an emergency? You just want to get to the hospital as soon as possible. Hospital CEOs want the hospitals to make as much money as possible. Profits at for-profit hospitals go to investors, and profits at nonprofit hospitals are hidden in a maze of accounting tricks. The patient becomes the captive. One of my patients calls this extortion "pay up or die."

Executives, many of whom are not MDs, handling a part of the $4 trillion health care industry feel entitled to some of this gold mine. This includes building in a profit margin (even in nonprofit hospitals), high compensation for hospital administrators, and spendthrift enlargement of support staff. Many hospital CEOs (called hospital directors in the old days) are paid salaries of $1 million to $6 million. An army of senior executives are also paid excessively. Sutter Health System (nonprofit) have 22 executives paid more than $1 million a year. At the same time, I have cared for homeless persons who were bankrupted because of hospital bills.

Inefficiency and redundancy in hospitals largely result from the monopoly business model. Teams of doctors and nurses are hired to write moneymaking protocols. Employees are dedicated to squeezing dollars from insurance companies. I have talked to administrators who spend all day, every day in meetings. I once asked an administrator, "What did you accomplish yesterday?" The response: "I just went to eight meetings." Who pays for administrators to sit through meetings? Working American families pay directly or indirectly (box 2.2).

In addition, too many hospitals have engaged in building and remodeling projects to create a grand hotel or Disneyland atmosphere. Building new structures that may only be used a few hours a day drives up health care costs.

Evolution of the Corporate Business Model: Deceptions That Increase Hospital Revenue

Total hospital costs represent over 30% of the US health care dollar, about $4,000 for each man, woman, and child in this country. I once defended outrageous hospital pricing. I was the front man and spokes-

Box 2.2

To fully understand this chapter, knowledge of one of the federal government systems of paying for medical care is important. More details on these programs are discussed in chapter 4, "Health Plans." In a nutshell, the fee schedules used by Medicare control costs and, if adapted universally, would help contain overall health care costs in America.

This federal health care program is for people aged 65 and over and any age with certain medical conditions, such as kidney failure requiring dialysis. It pays a set fee to doctors, based on the complexity of care rendered, and a set fee to the hospital. In order not to be nickeled and dimed by the hospital for every band aid, nurse visit, IV start, or special meal, Medicare requires that charges be bundled by diagnostic rate group (DRG). For example, if a person is admitted for a hip replacement, the hip replacement DRG might be $40,000 versus the list price of individually tallied items of $100,000. Medicare will pay $40,000, and no more. The patient cannot be balance billed for any amount that Medicare does not pay. Balanced billing can occur when a person receives care by an out-of-network physician or hospital and it obligates the person to pay out of pocket the difference between any insurance payment and the full retail list price by the hospital. Medicare's prohibition of balanced billing is an important protection for its members.

You might think, does the hospital eat a $60,000 loss for each hip replacement in a Medicare patient? No! Medicare conducts periodical audits of hospital costs to delivery service. This varies by location because of differing labor and other hospital costs. In the case of the $35,000 they get for a hip replacement, it may have only cost them $30,000. They still make a profit.

person for unbelievably high ED charges as chief of emergency medicine at University of California, Davis. I remember a live broadcast interview in the 1990s with *ABC News* anchor Sam Donaldson. It took place in the ED where I sat on a high stool with lights glaring in my face with ED patients and noise in the background. We talked via videoconferencing on huge TV screens. Donaldson kept asking how our hospital could bill $20 for a two-cent tablet of acetaminophen (Tylenol). I defended the hospital, using the standard excuse of high charges to cover the cost of caring for uninsured patients. I was wrong and regret what I said in the interview. What would I say now? "The hospital is greedy and wants to make a high profit. It has built in inefficiencies, with a bloated number of staff, and overcharges health plans. Sadly, some patients get caught in the middle, paying $20 out of pocket for a single Tylenol tablet." Some deceptions hospitals employ to increase revenue follow:

1. *Monopoly price gouging for hospital care.* Hospitals are run like businesses that have a monopoly, and they set retail prices to maximize profit. As a rule of thumb, hospitals charge two to three times and sometimes more above the actual cost. Prices, if listed at all, are not posted in an easy, accessible, and understandable way to the public. I used the following example in speeches I made when I ran for Congress in 2016, "The hospital business model is like going into a grocery store that does not post grocery prices, picking up a half-gallon of milk and then 60 days later receiving a bill for $100. Would any of us tolerate that? No. Then why do we tolerate that behavior from hospitals?" After reading this book, the reader will understand and be motivated to help make change.

We see many examples of outrageous hospital charges for medical treatment in the news media. I could fill pages of this book with examples, as well as the stories my patients have told me directly.

One of the most powerful examples of outrageous pricing was described in Elizabeth Rosenthal, MD's, book *An American Sickness.* Dr. Rosenthal describes an uninsured woman who was hospitalized at the University of Virginia for a brain hemorrhage and received bills for nearly $320,000. In a nutshell, had the patient been covered by Medicare, it would have paid the hospital between $65,000 and $80,000, closer to the actual cost of care. The reader may find both the behavior and the pricing structure of the hospital in this case appalling.

So are hospitals taking a huge loss on Medicare patients? No, they aggressively compete for these patients, as I will describe later in this chapter.

2. *The culture of secret prices: the charge master.* Let's look at some hospital billing practices. Hospitals use an itemized master list of all services and items that it charges to bill health plans and

patients. This master list is called a *charge master* and is used to apply charges for any hospital services, including ED visits, outpatient services, operating room time, and inpatient hospitalization. The lists can be several thousand items long. Some states require posting of this list, in whole or in part, but many times, it is written in difficult-to-understand code and is confusing to find on the internet. Using code numbers and or unintelligible abbreviations for charges may be standard in billing health plans, but for most patients, it is not helpful in determining the real price. The federal government recently required posting some prices, but this is not helpful for determining true prices. How can a person know how many bandages they will be charged for? I favor preset prices, based on diagnosis, called diagnostic related groups, or DRGs. In other words, if a person is admitted for a heart attack, they are not nickeled and dimed for every item or service but pay a fixed price for the heart attack DRG. Sort of like a French restaurant prix fixe menu.

3. *Different rates for different folks: it's the out-of-pocket costs that hurt.* Let's look at hypothetical hospital charges for John Smith. In 2015, John was bitten by a poisonous rattlesnake and taken to a hospital ED where he was hospitalized for four days (yes, this is based on a true story). The hospital charges and his out-of-pocket debt could vary widely, depending on his insurance status.

a. Full retail charge: If John has no insurance, he is stuck paying the charge master rate (retail rate)—the full $100,000—out of pocket.

b. Full retail charge despite a health plan (insurance): If John's health plan does not have a contract with the hospital, the hospital will still send a bill for the full retail price of $100,000. The insurance company may pay less than the $100,000, claiming that under the term "reasonable and customary," the $100,000 is too much. If John's health plan pays only $50,000, then John is stuck with $50,000 out of pocket.

c. Discounted rate: Many health plans have contracts with the in-network hospitals. The discounted rate for the rattlesnake bite example could be $60,000, $40,000 less than the $100,000 retail rate.

Because of the contract, John cannot be billed for the balance of $40,000. Most health plans then pay 80% of the $60,000, leaving John to pay the remaining 20% of the $60,000. So John's out of pocket is $12,000, unless he has a plan with a lower maximum annual deductible.

d. Federal and state programs: Medicare and Medicaid programs require the hospital to take a set rate; John will not have to pay the balance. Using the snakebite example, the maximum allowable charge under Medicare might be $35,000. John's out-of-pocket expense would be the Medicare deductible (currently $1,300) for inpatient hospital care. Since Medicare considers treatments that occurred in the ED as an outpatient charge, he would also owe the hospital 20% of Medicare allowable ED charges. Since most Medicare beneficiaries also have private secondary insurance, out-of-pocket charges could be as low as a few hundred dollars. Minimal out-of-pocket charges are a major reason why many members of the US Congress favor Medicare for all.

e. Other programs: Other iterations of charges and out-of-pocket costs exist. Some HMOs, for example, Kaiser Permanente health systems, may rescue its members if they seek emergency care at a non–Kaiser facility, by sending an ambulance to move them to a Kaiser facility. Patients may have limited out-of-pocket costs in true emergencies. Kaiser may or may not have contracts with other facilities, and I have heard that trauma centers gouge Kaiser to increase their bottom line.

4. *Billing errors that benefit the hospital: another means of cheating patients?* The September 2018 issue of *Consumer Reports* described hospital-billing practices, including errors. One example cited a 32-year-old man with a $33,000 bill from Dignity Northridge Hospital in California. His health care insurance should have covered the cost. Somehow, the hospital messed up the billing, and because they did not receive payment, the full bill was sent to the patient. His account was sent to a collection agency, and it took nearly two years to straighten things out. My patients have told countless stories about billing errors and major fights to prevent hospitals from cheating them, resulting in emotional distress, sleepless nights, and financial worries.

5. *Sending your account to a collection agency.* On June 5, 2016, HBO's *Last Week Tonight with John Oliver* investigated the debt-buying industry. Oliver was able to buy nearly $15 million in medical debt for less than a penny on the dollar. For $60,000, he bought the debt of 9,000 people who owed money and then forgave them all. Some hospitals set up payment plans for patients that don't have cash on hand. However, unethical hospitals may "sell" this debt to a collection agency. In some cases, patient debt is sold for pennies on the dollar. But they won't transfer the same pennies-on-the-dollar relief to their patients.

6. *Outright fraud.* In fiscal year 2017, the Department of Health and Human Services and the Department of Justice recovered $2.6 billion from judgments, settlements, and additional impositions in health care fraud cases and proceedings. This is consistent with other recent years, with billions of dollars accessed as a result of medical fraud. Many of these settlements, some in the hundreds of millions of dollars, were due to fraud committed by hospitals and national hospital chains. The recoveries were attributable partially to the work of the Health Care Fraud and Abuse Control Program, which is designed to coordinate federal, state, and local law enforcement activities to combat health care fraud. Using 2017 as an example, the DOJ opened 967 new criminal health care fraud investigations, and federal prosecutors filed criminal charges in 439 cases involving 720 defendants. A total of 639 defendants were convicted of health care fraud–related crimes in fiscal year 2017. A few examples have been selected from hundreds of settlements from alleged illegal activities committed by hospitals over the years:

a. 2018: Prime Healthcare Services, Inc agreed to pay the United States $65 million to settle allegations that 14 Prime hospitals in California knowingly submitted false claims to Medicare by admitting patients who required only less costly, outpatient care and by billing for more expensive patient diagnoses than the patients had (a practice known as "up-coding"), the Justice Department announced today. Under the settlement agreement, Prime will pay $61,750,000 (https://www.justice.gov/opa/pr/prime-healthcare-services-and-ceo-pay-65-million-settle-false-claims-act-allegations).

b. 2018: William Beaumont Hospital, a regional hospital system based in the Detroit, Michigan area, will pay $84.5 million to resolve allegations under the False Claims Act of improper relationships with eight referring physicians, resulting in the submission of false claims to the Medicare, Medicaid and TRICARE programs, the Justice Department announced today (https://www.justice.gov/opa/pr/detroit-area-hospital-system-pay-845-million-settle-false-claims-act-allegations-arising).

c. 2016: A major United States hospital chain, Tenet Healthcare Corporation, and two of its Atlanta-area subsidiaries will pay over $513 million to resolve criminal charges and civil claims relating to a scheme to defraud the United States and to pay kickbacks in exchange for patient referrals (https://www.justice.gov/opa/pr/hospital-chain-will-pay-over-513-million-defrauding-united-states-and-making-illegal-payments).

d. 2015: The Department of Justice has reached 70 settlements involving 457 hospitals in 43 states for more than $250 million related to cardiac devices that were implanted in Medicare patients in violation of Medicare coverage requirements, the Department of Justice announced today. Medicare coverage for the device, which costs approximately $25,000, is governed by a National Coverage Determination (NCD) (https://www.justice.gov/opa/pr/nearly-500-hospitals-pay-united-states-more-250-million-resolve-false-claims-act-allegations).

e. 2014: The Justice Department announced today that Community Health Systems Inc. (CHS), the nation's largest operator of acute care hospitals, has agreed to pay $98.15 million to resolve multiple lawsuits alleging that the company knowingly billed government health care programs for inpatient services that should have been billed as outpatient or observation services. The settlement also resolves allegations that one of the company's affiliated hospitals, Laredo Medical Center (LMC), improperly billed the Medicare program for certain inpatient procedures and for services rendered to patients referred in violation of the Physician Self-Referral Law, commonly known as the Stark Law. CHS is based in Franklin, Tennessee, and has 206 affiliated hospitals in 29 states (https://www .justice.gov/opa/pr/community-health-systems-inc-pay-9815-million -resolve-false-claims-act-allegations).

An even larger settlement of $260 million occurred with a hospital chain run by Health Management Associates in 2018. I encourage the reader to read the many examples of hospital fraud listed on the DOJ webpages.

7. *Making physicians do what is best for hospitals' bottom line, not what is best for the patients.* Hospitals' rules of operation were historically founded on the principle of physician control. Each hospital in the United States had a medical staff executive committee, which made rules on physician conduct and certified that physicians who treated hospital patients were competent and qualified. In addition, the committee, through its elected physician chairperson, the chief of staff, ensured that the hospital director (now called CEO) managed the hospital in the best interests of its patients.

That has changed. While medical staff committees still exist, now many hospital administrators attempt to tell physicians what they should be doing and how they should practice medicine. In my opinion this "MBA" method of management of hospitals places profit ahead of patient safety. Some hospitals even have physicians sign loyalty oaths, whereby the physician promises to do what the administration tells them to do, and not what is best for patients. If you do not sign, then you lose your privileges to care for patients in that hospital.

The DOJ announced that Community Health System would pay $98 million to resolve False Claims Act allegations. Emergency physicians claimed they were forced to admit patients to hospitals that did not need admission and order unneeded laboratory studies. Forcing physicians to admit patients to increase hospital profits was a focus of "Hospitals: The Cost of Admission" on CBS's *60 Minutes* on December 3, 2012.

An example of doctors fighting a corporate type of takeover and non-physician control of safety rules occurred in 2016, at the

Tulare, California, Regional Medical Center (TRMC). The board of directors (elected laypersons), encouraged by the hospital administration, voted to terminate physician members of the hospital's medical staff committee. This would effectively remove the hospital's elected medical staff officers, allow the administration to appoint their own officers, and approve new rules drafted without physician input. Many physicians had privileges terminated and were stripped of their rights as active members. Physicians enlisted the help of the California Medical Association (CMA). A legal battle between the physicians and hospital ensued. A settlement was reached which fully reinstated the medical staff, its officers and bylaws.

8. *Prolonging pain and suffering in the ED.* So many hospitals advertise excellence in patient care, or something along those lines. Yet they turn a blind eye to their EDs, where patients wait hours to be seen by a physician. Sick and admitted patients stack up in crowded hallways, while patients admitted for high-profit elective procedures have no delays in obtaining a hospital bed. This problem will be discussed in detail in chapter 7 ("Emergency Departments").

9. *Increasing monopolies by squeezing or closing rural hospitals.* Large hospital systems may buy up small rural hospitals that serve an essential service to local communities. The mega system will then slowly close down some or all of the services provided by the rural hospital, leaving the patients no choice but to go to the nearest big town or small city. A 10-minute drive to the hospital becomes an hours-long commute to get care in a neighboring city or town. The nearest open hospital may be owned by the hospital system that closed down the rural hospital. For example, the giant Sutter Health System bought the Del Norte District Hospital in Crescent City (pop. 7,000). It faced local community opposition when it attempted to reduce hospital services and size from 49 to 25 beds. A lawsuit by the local community resulted in a settlement to maintain the hospital capacity of 49 beds.

10. *Observational status: more out-of-pocket costs for Medicare recipients.* Sometimes people may be hospitalized for several days but will not be classified as inpatient admissions. Instead, patients are

classified under *observational status*. This means that health plans and Medicare consider all treatments, procedures, drugs, and imaging as outpatient services. Observation status may be applied to patients even if they are hospitalized for injuries with multiple broken bones or for pneumonia that requires IV drugs. This increases costs for patients. Hospitals claim that Medicare rules that define criteria for real admission are so limiting that hospitals use observational status to avoid Medicare fines. These rules were implemented to prevent fraudulent admissions. A hypothetical example of a fraudulent admission would be admitting someone to the hospital for an ankle sprain. But on the flip side, not hospitalizing or delaying by several hours a person who needs hospitalization will result in higher fees, as ED fees may generate more profit than inpatient fees.

Some consumer advocates claim that hospitals make more money by charging for every service, pill, or bandage, instead of charging a single bundled payment for a DRG, used by Medicare and some health plans for true inpatient admissions.

Patients with Medicare cannot have rehabilitation services at a nursing home paid by Medicare if they have been hospitalized under "observational status."

Solutions: Breaking Up the Hospital Monopoly Business Model

1. *Federal Campaign Finance Reform: outlaw campaign contributions to Congress by the hospital industry.* The majority of Americans believe that health care is a human right. Why are we selling our rights to the highest bidder? Similar to the problem discussed in chapter 1, "Prescription Drugs," the root cause of our health care problems is a political system that lets hospital corporations "buy" votes from the US Congress. Contributions to the election campaigns of both houses of Congress come with a string attached: the member of Congress gets money to get elected and then is "expected" to support legislation favorable to the industry. How can a US senator

or representative vote in the best interest of the people when future large contributions to their political campaigns depend on their voting in favor of corporate profits?

2. *Prohibit lobbying by the hospital industry.* Currently, nearly 1,000 professional lobbyists work for hospitals and hospital associations to influence Congress. These small armies of lobbyists descend on Congress, present their one-sided view of the health care system, and advocate for new rules and laws that benefit their financial bottom line.

Prohibiting lobbying by corporations and corporate groups would provide Congress a more objective view of health care through professional research, testimony by experts, input from the National Institutes of Health, and discussions with everyday Americans individually and at town halls. The result will be legislation that improves health care, not profits.

3. *Set maximum prices at the Medicare reimbursement level and end outrageous charges to patients.* Congress has the power to control monopolies. In 1906, Congress passed the Hepburn Act, which gave the federal government the power to set maximum prices that railroads could charge for freight. Now, more than 100 years later, hospital monopolies need regulation for the public good. A successful pricing system has already been established for Medicare patients. Medicare determines the rates it pays hospitals based on analysis of actual costs of delivering health care. It also includes a small profit. As a general rule of thumb, Medicare pays 30% to 50% of the hospital retail "list price." Medicare rates need to be applied to all patients using hospital services. Think of the enormous savings to our country if hospitals were prohibited from charging more than the Medicare rate. Oh, you might say this is against our free enterprise system. Wrong. Hospitals have monopolies, just like your electric utility, and just like a utility needs regulation to prevent price gouging, so should hospitals with monopolies have prices regulated.

4. *List the prices for care.* Confusing prices listed in a hospital's charge master do not tell the complete story about how much hospital care will actually cost. Would you buy a half-gallon of milk without

knowing the price? What if the store employee told you he did not know the price, but you would get a bill in the mail in a month? And what if that bill was for $1,000 for just a half-gallon of milk? Hospitals currently do not post the prices on their front door, or for that matter elsewhere in the hospital. I have been to hospitals overseas in which prices for common problems are posted outside the front door, and less common conditions are listed on a wall poster. Think of the choices we would have if, for example, prices were listed up front for the following conditions:

Chest pain evaluation in the ER: $200
Headache evaluation and treatment: $150
Suturing a small laceration on the hand: $195

5. *Enact criminal statutes that require jail time and fines for hospital administrators and executives that commit fraud.* Currently, CEOs and executives who direct policies that result in grossly unfair practices, cheating, and fraud rarely go to jail. Most hospital administrators involved in DOJ fraud settlements escape personal consequences. If they were held accountable and faced jail time, their motivation to direct unethical and illegal practices would be reduced.

6. *Enact and enforce a patient's financial bill of rights.* The September 2018 issue of *Consumer Reports* proposed a bill of rights for patients. Highlights of their proposal include:

1. the right to see a price list,
2. a prohibition on surprise medical bills from out-of-network physicians,
3. provide an up-front price estimate with maximum costs before service is rendered,
4. provide an itemized bill in simple layman terms.

Bottom line: Extreme hospital charges hurt the American family for the benefit of more profit for the hospital industry. As with prescription drugs, only the US Congress must solve this inequality through legislative actions.

THREE

Physicians

KEY CONCEPTS

1. Small office-based primary care has given way to hospital-based primary care.
2. Assembly-line corporate protocols have commandeered physicians' independent decision making.
3. Physicians may spend up to 50% of their time on computer data entry.
4. Bedside health care by primary care physicians has been eclipsed by fragmented care by multiple specialists.
5. Increasing numbers of nurse practitioners, physician assistants, and others are providing frontline medical care.

Health professionals' money spent on lobbying members of Congress in 2018: $91,000,000

Health professionals' campaign contributions in 2018: $70,859,000

My earliest memory of needing a good, caring doctor was when I fell onto a wooden staircase at my school playground, resulting in a huge splinter driven under one of my fingernails up and beyond the nail bed. It hurt like crazy. I needed medical care. I ran home, and my mom had me wait for my dad because she did not drive.

That evening, my dad took me to a public infirmary, not too far from our house. In Los Angeles in the 1950s, a scattering of these public clinics offered free care. Hardly anyone was in the waiting room, and I was taken right away, where a kind and gentle physician extracted the splinter, bandaged my finger, and sent us on our way.

Driving home I asked, "How much did that cost, Dad?"

"Nothing. It was free," he said.

"Wow, maybe I should become a doctor, and fix people for free," I said.

The first seed was sown in my mind that pushed me toward a career in medicine—at the young age of 10. (I dumped the thought of becoming a firefighter or jet fighter pilot.) So I went to college, graduated, and was accepted to several medical schools. The four years of medical school was one of the most enjoyable of my life; there was so much to learn and it was exciting. After graduating from medical school, I advanced to the next level of training.

All of my 135 fellow students and I went on to additional training called a *residency*. Some decided to specialize in family practice, general surgery, or pediatrics. A few chose surgical specialties, such as orthopedics; ear, nose, and throat; or urology. But most chose internal medicine. In the summer of 1975, I started my internship and residency at the University of California, Davis, teaching hospital in Sacramento, California.

I had waffled during my last two years of medical school about whether to become a surgeon or choose a path in internal medicine, such as primary care, cardiology, or infectious diseases. I loved my surgical rotations, and as a senior student, I served as "surgeon" for a simple abdominal operation called a laparotomy under the supervision of a second-year surgical resident. I loved surgery but instead applied for further training in internal medicine. Maybe my girlfriend, Jeannie, had a role, reminding me that surgeons wake up to an alarm at 5 o'clock every morning. But it explains why I ultimately became an ED doctor, so I could sleep in but still do some surgical procedures on shifts that began late.

Additional training for doctors takes three to five years after graduating from medical school, and sometimes even longer. After three years of my residency, I entered the world of medical practice. I decided to stay in an academic environment at UC Davis Medical Center in Sacramento and went to work in the ED, learning the new skills of emergency care on the job. But most of my colleagues went into "business," working in private practice, either in solo practices or with small groups of physicians. This cottage industry of small clusters of physicians functioning as independent small businesses formed the backbone of the health care delivery system at that time.

Independent private practice physicians had reasonable charges, did x-rays in the office, did simple lab work, and looked at your blood, urine, or sputum under their own microscope with their own eyes. Prior to the 1990s, health care insurance was inexpensive and generally paid for by the employer. Paying for doctor care was not a hardship, and many physicians would provide free care to those in need. In rural areas, a bill could be paid off with eggs, firewood, or field and yard work. Prescription drugs were cheap, and it was not uncommon for physicians to dispense medications for a nominal fee.

When a person became sick or injured and required hospitalization, the family doctor would go to the hospital to provide ongoing medical care. Today, this happens less and less. Besides making patients feel better because the doctor was familiar with the patient, the doctor could make better decisions regarding care and ordered fewer tests. Private hospital bills were less expensive and limited to a daily room charge and minimal costs of some supplies, lab, x-rays, and medications. Public hospitals and clinics served lower-income folks and generally charged minimal or no fee. Nearly every county and major city had a public hospital staffed by doctors in training with minimal supervision by attending physicians.

But the physician's office-based cottage industry was under attack by leading economists who felt that corporate assembly-line economies of scale would improve the quality and decrease the cost of medical care, which I learned when I attended a Harvard University short course for chiefs of major clinical services in January 1994. In addition to braving Boston's freezing temperatures, I learned that the delivery models of medical care in the United States had to be changed. The leading example used by the professor was that of a Danish furniture company that assembled furniture piece by piece, instead of using a corporate assembly line. The furniture company went broke: translation by the professor, the cottage industry of medical care had to change. I disagree. Unlike furniture, people cannot be healed by an assembly line.

So what did the cottage industry model of health care delivery look like for patients and physicians before Wall Street gained the upper hand? Here is a snapshot of the traditional cottage industry model of health care that offered one-stop shopping and efficiency.

A colleague of mine, Dr. Nayvin Gordon sums up primary care in the 1970s and 1980s:

Patients generally could get an appointment the same day. The office staff worked for me: My practice would sink or swim based on whom I hired or fired. I had complete control of my schedule. I could do simple x-rays in my office. So I would immediately know if there was an abnormality that needed intervention. I could do splinting and casting. I could suture wounds and perform a long list of procedures from injecting knees to draining abscesses. I had a microscope and could examine my patient's blood, urine, wound pus, and other samples. Thus, there was no waiting for a report from a laboratory and, in the case of x-rays, no delay in getting x-rays or waiting for a radiologist to look at the film. If I needed to refer one of my patients to a specialist, such as to a surgeon or a cancer physician, my staff could make a call and the patient was usually seen in a day or two. Then I would receive a telephone call or detailed letter regarding treatment recommendations for my patient. Some of my colleagues would dispense prescription drugs for a small fee. My charges were reasonable; the patients would first pay out of pocket, roughly $30 ($96 in today's dollars). The majority of people were reimbursed by their insurance company, perhaps leaving them on the hook for only a buck or two. But if you did not have money or insurance, the charges were often reduced or waived. If one of my patients needed hospitalization, I would be the doctor in charge of their care and see them every day, sometimes both in the morning as well as in the evening after my clinic closed. I did not need to order unnecessary testing or consultants in the hospital because I knew my patients well from years of caring for them in the practice. This primary care model offered the best bang for the buck. It was also fun, and I went to work every day happy; this created a positive experience for my patients. And, by the way, my $30 fee also had to pay for office staff salaries, equipment, rent, insurance, heating, and AC.

To better understand the changes in medicine from bedside care to corporate care, I want to first review the steps to become a practicing physician.

The Long Pathway to Become a Physician

This section is written to help my students and other readers better understand the steps required to become a practicing physician.

1. *College.* The first step is to do well in a four-year college or university in basic academics and meet the medical school application requirements that generally require courses in biology, chemistry, and physics. In addition, you have to score well on a national entrance exam called MCAT. Forty years ago, about one-in-four applicants ultimately were accepted to a US medical school, but this acceptance ratio has varied from one-in-two to one-in-five over this time span. More recently, extracurricular activities are taken into account, such as community service, research, and volunteer work at a clinic or other organization providing medical care.

2. *Medical school.* A four-year curriculum leads to a doctor of medicine (MD) degree. This four-year curriculum has undergone a number of minor changes but has remained similar in structure since the 1960s. The first two years involve classroom teaching, and the last two years require clinical rotations of one month or more with a group of physicians providing hospital care. By the time one finishes medical school, one will have spent time with specialty teams such as internal medicine, surgery, pediatrics, obstetrics and gynecology, orthopedics, family practice, among others. Medical education costs have exploded: I paid a $300-a-year student fee to attended UC San Francisco. Now it costs medical students $41,000 a year.

Osteopathic schools have similar curricula and costs but offer a doctor of osteopathy (DO) degree. DOs are equivalent to MDs, and some of our brightest ED residents are DOs. DOs are included as physicians in this book.

3. *Residency.* After completing medical school, newly minted doctors spend another three to six years in postdoctoral training called *residency*. Training beyond residency is often referred to as a *fellowship*. A residency provided bedside training in a teaching

hospital, supplemented with focused lectures. In the past, a newly minted physician would spend the first year in a rotating internship, moving month by month among different hospital specialty services. Only then would a new physician apply to specialty residencies, spending an additional two to four years in on-the-job training. Now the rotating internship is gone. Instead, after graduating from medical school, physicians go directly into one of nearly 20 specialties. A three-year family practice residency has replaced general practice. Residents in training earn about $60,000 a year.

4. *Medical licenses.* A medical license, granted by individual states, is required to practice medicine, and each state has its own requirements beyond medical school. Some states require one year of internship or residency; others require three years. A physician can practice only in the state in which he or she is licensed; for example, a California-licensed physician cannot practice in Nevada, unless she obtains a separate Nevada license. Although there is no federal license to prescribe certain medications, referred to as *controlled substances*, physicians must obtain a Drug Enforcement Agency (DEA) certificate, which must be renewed every three years.

5. *Board certification.* After completing a residency, physicians must pass an exam in their respective specialty to be awarded board certification. Before the 1980s, board certification was permanent, now it expires after 10 years. I took a written exam in internal medicine and was awarded a permanent certificate in 1978. In contrast, I took both an oral and a written exam in 1986 to become board certified in emergency medicine and needed to renew every 10 years, which I did through three 10-year cycles. How did I become board certified in emergency medicine without completing an ED residency? For the answer, read chapter 7, "Emergency Departments."

To renew certification, physicians must attend specific classes and pass another exam. Some specialties, such as internal medicine, have subspecialties, such as cardiology and infectious diseases, which require an additional two or more years of bedside training.

6. *Ongoing requirements.* To maintain both an active medical license and board certification, physicians participate in other activities. Examples include continuing medical education (CME) activities, and specific maintenance of board certification (MOC) requirements such as web-based online study guides and online exams. Hospitals may require additional mini-certificates, such as cardiopulmonary resuscitation (CPR), advanced trauma life support (ATLS), advanced cardiac life support (ACLS), and others. Averaged over several years these activities can cost more than $5,000 per year. Finally, many physicians need to register and update information with specific agencies, such as the Council for Affordable Quality Healthcare (CAQH), Controlled Substance Utilization Review and Evaluation System (CURES in California), as well as local medical societies.

From Independent Cottage Industry to Cog in the Corporate Assembly Line

Many of my colleagues would object to this subheading, but I am trying to make an important point. In the past, most physicians were self-employed or partners in small self-governing groups. At present, practice management or hospital corporations employ more and more physicians, including primary care physicians (PCPs), emergency physicians, anesthesiologists, radiologists, and hospitalists. Independence of physician thought—the key to good, individualized medical care—has slowly given way to protocols, unneeded testing, and procedures, driven by computer algorithms. When did the change occur? It was not sudden, and I would say began in the 1990s and mostly complete by 2020.

The old cottage industry was great for physicians and our patients. But insurance companies have made requirements for payment increasingly difficult and have reduced payments for PCPs. Now, relatively few primary care private practices of only one or two physicians survive, and for those that do, physicians work long hours for less pay than hospital-based physicians. Would a newly minted physician with

$300,000 in educational debt take a job for $75,000 a year as a solo practitioner or a corporate job that offers $200,000?

These few remaining solo or small-group primary care practices struggle to stay afloat. These physicians are truly dedicated to their Hippocratic oath of serving the public, working long hours, fighting billing companies and hospital bureaucracy, and taking home $75,000 or so a year. Contrast this to a surgeon caught sending a patient a bill for $117,000 for assisting just a few hours in a surgery (Rosenthal 2014).

The economies of scale model does not work for health care. Corporate models have moved health care delivery in the opposite direction, toward lower productivity for doctors and inconvenience and high fees for their patients. Problems range from inefficient computer demands, to rigid protocols, to fragmented medical care. Let's use grocery shopping as a metaphor for the issue of fragmented medical care. Imagine having to drive to six different stores to buy vegetables, milk, meat, cereal, bread, and canned goods. That's less efficient than a one-stop supermarket. What if each specialty food store source, such as a bakery, butcher shop, vegetable stand, or dairy, was located in a different city? My patients may routinely face this inefficiency, driving to an in-network diabetic specialist 50 miles away, when an out-of-network specialist is located a few miles from their home. And then add the extra time and inefficiency for me to try to get the medical report from out-of-town specialists.

Corporate Changes Affect Physicians and Patients

As a US congressional candidate, I talked to thousands of voters at town hall meetings and political events in 2015 and 2016. Many Americans still admire and expect the old "bedside medicine" model of health care delivery. People complained not only about high costs but that medical care had become impersonal, with physicians spending more time typing into a computer than looking at and listening to their patients in the examination room. I frequently listened to voters' concerns that they couldn't find a primary care doctor to take care of them.

They asked, "What are you going to do about that?" Well, I lost the election, and could not introduce legislation in Congress, so what I am doing is writing this book. Corporate changes to health care continue, and voters are angry.

From Small Primary Care Office to Hospital-Based Clinic

Sometime in the 1980s a progressive, step-by-step process began that resulted in today's corporate model of health care delivery. Most primary care practices are now part of a hospital group, an academic medical center, or a corporate-owned medical practice. What motivates physicians to join a hospital-based practice? Independent, small mom-and-pop offices are not financially viable for several reasons: (1) health plans pay much more to hospital-based clinics, (2) health plans reduce or deny payments to freestanding office practices, and (3) the multiple, expensive, and time-consuming bureaucratic requirements from health plans and governments are difficult for the individual to meet.

In traditional private practice, there is only one charge for an office visit called the *professional fee*. Say, the professional fee is $100. It must cover the doctor's pay, salary of office staff, office rent, utilities, insurance, and supplies and equipment. Hospitals lobbied Congress so that hospital-based clinics are able to charge an additional fee called the *facility use fee,* as well as a professional fee. A hospital-based clinic can charge the $100 professional fee (billed in the doctor's name) plus a facility use fee upward of $300. Business managers run hospital-based clinics and, in my opinion, are more interested in the bottom line than the patient welfare. Doctors may have little or no say in hiring or firing staff. Loss of control of scheduling of patients can result in longer wait times for patients, bottlenecks during the day, and overall frustration for both patients and physicians. Clinic administrators add productivity demands on physicians regarding number of patients seen per day and relative effort involved, measured by the relative value unit (RVU). (A deeper discussion can be found in the section "The

Growth of Specialists" in this chapter.) The key measure of good doctors can now be how many RVUs per hour they generate, not how well their patients like them.

Other factors also cause small practices to close and force physicians into hospital-based clinics. In the late 1980s and 1990s, health plans accelerated a practice of arbitrarily reducing payment for services or flat-out denying payment. Surgeons who submitted a usual and customary fee of $1,000 for an appendectomy would be told their service is only worth $500. Primary care physicians were told that an office visit was unnecessary, even though a patient was seriously ill. Health plans would refuse to pay for laboratory tests the treating physician deemed necessary.

Hospital-based clinics have also eliminated many traditional "bedside" procedures performed by doctors. For example, examining patients' blood or urine samples under a microscope in real time allowed the doctor to better connect patients' symptoms with subtle lab findings and arrive at an accurate diagnosis. In the past, x-rays were more commonly done in physicians' offices. An enhanced appreciation of a patient's problem occurs when the examining physician views an x-ray with the patient in the examination room. This connection with the patient improved job pleasure. The loss of real-time laboratories is not entirely a result of corporate lobbying but, paradoxically, physician lobbying. Pathology specialists were the major force in getting Congress to pass the Clinical Laboratory Improvement Amendments of 1988. This law placed major roadblocks in office-based real-time analysis of patient blood, urine, and other samples. (See chapter 9, "Tests and Studies.")

Fewer Primary Care Physicians Take Care of Their Hospitalized Patients

Only a physician can admit a patient to the hospital. To admit a patient, the physician must have admitting privileges and have undergone a rigorous review by a hospital committee. In the past, a person's office-based PCP (e.g., family practice, internal medicine, pediatric, or general practice physician) admitted a patient to the hospital and provided ongoing care in the hospital, examining their patients once or twice a day, and writing treatment orders. Surgical specialists admitted patients for surgical procedures and also provided consultation to inpatients with surgical problems. Emergency department physicians cannot admit sick and injured patients to the hospital from the ED; they must call a physician with admitting privileges.

A physician called a hospitalist now admits most patients from the ED. The term *hospitalist* is new, commonly meaning a physician who admits and provides care to hospitalized patients. Hospitalists are trained in internal medicine. Rarely now does a PCP admit a patient directly from an office, calling the nursing floor with orders. Patients are now sent to the ED from office-based practices. If the person needs an urgent admission, for example, for pneumonia, the patient is most likely admitted by the hospitalist. The driving forces of this change are many and include (1) low fees (or even no fee) paid by the health plans to PCPs who care for hospitalized patients, (2) excessive demands by hospitals for PCPs to maintain admitting privileges, and (3) excessive time spent inputting office visits into a computer.

Continuity of care is lost and care becomes impersonal in the hospitalist system. Hospitalists usually work 12-hour shifts and after 12 hours hand off care to the next oncoming hospitalist. A person may see five different hospitalists in just a three-day stay. Each new hospitalist may have to ask the same set of redundant questions, adding to the inefficiency of health care. On the flip side, hospitalist work is difficult. In addition to learning about many brand-new patients each shift, they must integrate symptoms and physical exam findings with complex laboratory studies and radiologic imaging. And their services cost more than the traditional PCP who provided bedside hospital care. I spoke to a woman in my clinic who was hospitalized for three days on the obstetrics floor who told me several different hospitalists poked their heads in her hospital room and did nothing other than say hello. She received a bill for $6,000 from the hospitalists' employer, a Wall Street corporation.

The Electronic Medical Record

Computers now dominate nearly every aspect of medical care. The first thing I do after arriving in my medical office is to turn on the computer. I look at a long list of notifications, directing me to make addendums to medical records. Some are scolding notifications for various "failures": not entering the proper ICD-10 code, not providing a patient an immunization (computer wrong), not ordering lab tests on a patient with a certain condition (computer wrong), or ordering a medication the patient is allergic to (computer wrong again). Why, as the doctor, should I spend 10 minutes searching Google to find an ICD-10 code? What a waste of time. Sadly, many physicians prioritize data entry over patient interaction.

Health plans many years ago demanded electronic medical records as part of an agreement to pay doctors. If physicians did not comply, they would receive less money for the visit. Congress cemented this concept by passing the Health Information Technology for Economic and Clinical Health (HITECH) Act of 2009, requiring electronic medical records (referred to as EHR or EMR). A physician who wants to get fully paid by a government health plan has to comply with HITECH regulations. The federal government provides a few dollars to help practices buy or lease computer software and hardware. The big institutions are able to buy advanced software, but smaller practices can only afford clunky, slow, and inefficient computer software. Extra time is required for physicians to enter the data. Pop-up boxes on the computer screens create roadblocks and detours that eat up valuable physician time. The extra time needed to navigate and enter data into computer systems has resulted in inefficiency. One physician recently told me that "in the old days I was 100% doctor. Now I am 40% doctor and 60% data entry clerk." Writing a prescription might take 15 minutes for three drugs versus 3 minutes on a handwritten prescription pad. Doctors who could see 30 patients a day before computers now see 20 a day. Doctors' eyes in many cases are glued to the computer screen and not on the patient. I once wrote an electronic prescription for migraine medication. The only way I could get the computer to transmit the prescription to the pharmacy was to provide a diagnosis of "migraine in second trimester." The pharmacist called an hour later to ask how a 60-year-old man could be pregnant.

Computer demands, as well as making RVU quotas, take away the most valuable asset of the physician—time to think. The added demands by the EHR can cause physicians to lose their perspective on the patient's real problem. I reviewed an ED malpractice case in which the real diagnosis was missed because the ED doctor and staff were so focused on correctly answering dumb questions required by the computer. In that case, an abdominal cancer was missed even though it was seen on imaging in the ED. Instead, the staff spent their time answering these questions:

Is the patient homeless?
Does the patient use barrier protection during sex?
Is the patient a fall risk?
Does the patient use seat belts?
Does the patient eat pizza more than twice a week?
How many alcohol drinks per week?
Has the patient experienced domestic abuse?
Has the patient ever been depressed?

By the time the staff was done with the questions, there was no time to thoroughly read the radiologist's report describing an abnormal mass. Who is to blame for the error that occurred in this medical malpractice case? It is the ominous burdens of the EHR that we can trace back to the HITECH Act, health plans that lobbied for it, and the Congress that voted for it. The HITECH Act and other federal legislation have added loads of additional data that get in the way of taking care of a patient's needs. Using the needle-in-a-haystack metaphor, imagine the needle is the diagnosis and treatment. Each piece of straw— the computer-mandated questions—covers the needle more and more. Enough pieces of straw hide the needle. The straw actually has an official term called *meaningful use*. This term is doublespeak, a term coined by author George Orwell in his book *1984*.

Meaningful use has also increased medical errors. Clicking quickly here and there on the EMR sometimes leads to clicking the wrong box. Demand for extra information wastes time and can be flat-out wrong, diverting attention from solving the real problem.

Corporate protocols are frequently embedded within the EMR. The EMR computer screen may flash pop-up boxes telling the physician what they should or should not order. Has the computer smelled the patient? Has it looked at or examined the patient? No. A few subtle cues that can be picked up by the physician may not be accepted as data by the computer. Then there are also EMR detectives that now track what a doctor did or did not do. How many flu vaccines did the physician order? How many colonoscopies? Was oseltamivir prescribed when flu was diagnosed? If physicians do not meet the corporate standard, they may receive less pay, a reprimand, or even be fired. *The danger occurs when a corporation has interest in pushing a drug or vaccine that might be harmful to certain patients.*

The Growth of Specialists

One of my patients came to see me solely because her insurance said she needed a primary care doctor. Each ailment had an assigned specialist:

Type 2 diabetes: endocrinologist
Chronic obstructive pulmonary disease (COPD): pulmonary specialist
Coronary artery disease (CAD): cardiologist
Migraine headaches: neurologist
Back pain: pain specialist
Sun damage: dermatologist

She told me she was on "lots of medicines" but could only recall the names of a few and did not know the doses of these. I had no access to the medical records from all her specialists. Sadly, this is too common. A good primary care practice could handle all these problems.

In fact, on subsequent visits, I discontinued or adjusted doses of her prescription medications. Many had dangerous interactions from the piecemeal prescribing from half a dozen physicians. How did we get here?

In the past, the family doctor would perform surgery, in most cases minor, but in some cases major. I even talked to a rural GP Idaho physician who implanted artificial hip joints. Back in 1950, 50% of physicians were listed as general practice physicians. Plus a number of general internists provided primary care. Now only about 10% of physicians are listed as general or family practice. And many internal medicine specialists (internists) have received additional training to become specialized in procedure-oriented disciplines, such as cardiology and gastroenterology. Fees collected from performing procedures are generous.

Specialists have performed miracles with advanced special procedures and improved the quality of life for millions of people but at a price. This list of procedures would cover several pages of this book but most commonly recognized are colonoscopy, cardiac cauterization, and cataract surgery. Procedures can help in two ways: to restore health (e.g., eyesight) or to diagnose a problem (e.g., finding an ulcer with endoscopy). Many of my patients were nearly crippled and using crutches before having a knee replacement that allowed them to walk normally again.

However, studies have shown that these high-cost and sometimes moneymaking procedures are not always needed. Colonoscopy, a procedure used primarily to screen for colon cancer, has increased the incomes of gastroenterologists. In addition to the professional fee the doctor charges, the hospital or surgical center makes large amounts of money from the procedure by charging a facility use fee.

Debate has been ongoing among PCPs and specialists regarding income and who works harder. The reader of this book may be shocked to learn that specialists make very high incomes, far more than PCPs. For example, a typical PCP makes about $180,000 to $200,000 per year versus $375,000 for radiologists and $450,000 for orthopedic surgeons. A colleague of mine once said, "As a PCP, I need to know every-

Table 3.1. Examples of physician salaries in 2016

Physician	Salary
Orthopedic surgeon	$443,000
Radiologist	$375,000
Emergency department	$332,000
Family practice	$207,000
Pediatrician	$204,000

Source: From Medscape, https://www.medscape.com.

thing about 100 dangerous drugs to earn my $180,000 a year. That's not fair, because an anesthesiologist only deals with 10 drugs, makes $350,000 a year, and then gets to go home after lunch" (table 3.1).

That opinion may not be shared by all PCPs, but it makes a point.

Why do specialists get paid more? It has little to do with their work ethic, intelligence, or knowledge. It's political. In the 1970s, relative value units, or RVUs, were derived primarily with influence from the American Medical Association. Specialists were well represented and made sure RVUs weighted heavily toward procedures. An RVU for a complex primary care visit (level 5) is 2.11, could take an hour, and could present very high stress for a physician racking their brains to make a diagnosis and derive a treatment plan. Contrast that with relocating a shoulder in the ED, which I've done many times. A shoulder relocation gets an RVU of 4.11, which may take only five minutes and can be as easy as pie, done at the same time the doctor is talking to the nurse about the next vacation to a tropical beach. (Sorry, I'm guilty of that.) Corporate managers also encourage physicians to increase their RVUs by seeing more patients or up-coding, that is, bumping up the visit to one that is more complex and pays a higher RVU.

The Network Puzzle: Doctor, Are You In Network or Out of Network?

The terms *in-network* and *out-of-network physicians* are a recent corporate invention. In network means the doctor has a contract with the health plan to accept a predefined fee per visit, usually at a discount. An out-of-network physician has no contract and is free to set the fee at any amount. Health plans may or may not pay the full fee for out-of-network visits. Or they may pay only a small fraction of the fee.

How does the ordinary person know who is in network? Health plans provide a list, which is in a constant state of flux. You might say, I'll be careful when choosing who provides me my medical care. But what if a person is already in a hospital bed at an in-network hospital? The person may have no choice of doctor who provides care and could get stuck with a big bill from an out-of-network physician. Out-of-network as well as in-network physicians can work at in-network hospitals.

In an emergency, a patient can be directed to an in-network hospital only to be seen by an out-of-network ED doctor. Or even if the ED physician is in network, the radiologist who reads the x-ray can be out of network. This also happens with elective surgery: the surgeon can be in network, but the anesthesiologist is out of network and sends a big charge for anesthesia, which the patient's health plan refuses to pay. A patient can be billed a fee for an out-of-network assistant surgeon that they have never talked with.

Jim B. (real name protected), a 62-year-old patient of mine, told me he was "ripped off." He received approval (after endless phone calls and submission of paperwork) from his employer-based health plan to have his knee replaced. Both the hospital and orthopedic surgeon were in network and thus accepted the health plan fee schedule. John researched co-pays and deductibles and was prepared to pay about $4,500 out of pocket. But a few weeks after surgery, he received an additional bill from an anesthesiology group for an additional $1,450, boosting his total out of pocket to nearly $6,000. He did not have the money, and now pays over 20% interest on this total on his credit card.

Jim's fee from the anesthesiology group is referred to as a *surprise medical bill*. I am not alone in hearing about these types of frustrations from patients. Out-of-network surprise medical bills have been the topic of discussion in professional publications. Traditional media such as newspapers and television as well as web-based media have published stories describing the unfairness of surprise medical bills. Some states have outlawed surprise medical bills. In California, emergency physicians can charge out-of-network patients only 125% of the Medicare pay rate. However, the process is not simple. One patient told me she had to hire an attorney at her own expense to get the ED physician management corporation to follow the rules.

The problem of surprise medical bills have reached the US Congress. In late spring of 2019, legislation was proposed by several members of Congress to address the issue, with S. 1531—Stopping the Outrageous Practice of Surprise Medical Bills Act of 2019. Corporate practice management groups that would risk decreased profits have launched a major attack against S. 1531, spending millions of dollars. As of the publication of this book, the fate of this legislation is unknown.

Add-On Physician Fees

Ever fly in a commercial aircraft? Not too long ago, the charge to fly economy from San Francisco to New York was a set dollar amount, for example, $500. Now it can be less than $400, plus a baggage fee, an extra leg room fee, onboard food, a pillow fee, and so forth, which can far exceed $500. Some doctors follow this moneymaking tactic; oncologists can add an infusion fee to give an IV drug. Even ED doctors can add a drug infusion fee and charge extra fees to clean blood off a wound (debridement) or to take a deep look into a person's throat (ICD code 529.0). Many doctors are in the top 5% income bracket. Why do they want more?

Medical Corporations Muzzle Doctors

The change from self-employed or small-group physician partnerships to physicians who work at corporate facilities has muzzled physicians who seek to provide the best care to their patients. An ED physician at a very busy Florida emergency department, who complained of severe overcrowding and asked for additional staffing, was fired. She alleges that she was fired because she complained about low ED staffing levels. A Missouri physician alleges she was fired for complaining about hospital safety issues. The American Academy of Emergency

Medicine has discussed physician termination and due process in many issues of its journal *Common Sense*. I have personally talked with physicians who were dismissed for complaining about unsafe patient environments.

Fear of Medical Malpractice Lawsuits

Many physicians who are employed by corporate entities worry they might lose their jobs if a successful malpractice lawsuit occurs and they lose in court, or are forced to settle. Do physicians order extra laboratory work, x-rays, and imaging and make unneeded referrals to specialists because they fear malpractice lawsuits? Yes, according to a recent study, which found that fear of a lawsuit was the reason that 84% of physicians ordered unneeded studies and treatment. This is especially true if they did not follow corporate written guidelines and algorithms. Most physicians who are employed by corporate entities have their malpractice premiums paid by the employer. US Congressman Ami Bera co-sponsored bill H.R. 4106 in 2014 that would provide protection from lawsuits provided established clinical guidelines were followed. The proposed legislation never progressed to a full House vote.

Nurse Practitioners and Physician Assistants

Although this chapter is about physicians, it would be incomplete if it did not mention that clinical care is also delivered by nurse practitioners (NPs) and physician assistants (PAs). In some rural areas, half the "doctoring" in primary care clinics may be provided by PAs and NPs. Their areas of practice have also expanded to EDs, hospital inpatient care, and specialist offices. States have different legal requirements regarding the degree of supervision and review by physicians. I have not researched the peer-reviewed literature of health care delivery by NPs and PAs. However, I can give you a personal opinion based on my experience. I have found that this group is very good at providing primary care but believe close supervision is needed in EDs.

Actions to Improve Doctor and Patient Satisfaction

As with other components of the health care system, change must be legislated through Congress. Lobbying by physician groups, such as the American Medical Association and physician professional societies, must focus on patient care issues, not physician pocketbook issues. Throw out the lobbyist who talks about reimbursement rates, and usher in physicians who are concerned about patient care, including cost of care to patients. Some specific steps to take include the following:

1. Help keep independent primary care practices open by requiring health plans and government plans to pay a facility use fee.
2. Put the doctor back in charge of the office, not the accountant, business manager, or Wall Street corporate CEO.
3. In corporate-owned practices, impose mandatory criminal fines and jail time to hospital or corporate heads that fire physicians who simply complain about problems related to delivery of care.
4. The federal government should provide tuition-free education at medical schools and, in return, require physicians to accept Medicare rates for providing medical and surgical care.
5. To help prevent Medicare fraud, cap the total dollars per year Medicare can pay individual physicians.
6. Revise Current Procedural Terminology (CPT) and RVU codes to benefit primary care physicians. Decrease RVUs and payments for procedures and interpretations of tests such as CT scans, x-rays, EKGs, and laboratory tests.
7. Prohibit add-on fees in hospital-based clinics such as supervision of IV infusions. This is a normal nurse function covered by the facility use fee.
8. Provide medical practices with simplified electronic health record software and computers for Electronic Medical Records (EHRs) free of charge and allow physicians to modify these as needed to increase efficiency. Eliminate the requirement

to enter redundant data such as requiring a reason for a prescription when the diagnosis provides that reason.

9. Revise the HITECH Act, including eliminating the "meaningful use provisions."
10. End the in-network versus out-of-network confusion with standardized national fee schedules, as done in most European countries.

Bottom line: Compassionate and personalized medical care is best delivered by caring physicians independent from the rules and regulations of corporate organizations. Congress must enact legislation that provides the financial and legal support needed to protect and sustain independent medical practice and thought.

[FOUR]

Health Plans

The Money Middlemen

KEY CONCEPTS

1. Most US health plans spend only 80% of revenue on actual health care and keep the rest for themselves.
2. In contrast, the US Medicare program and European health insurance plans spend 95% to 97% of revenue on health care.
3. Health plans limit choice of physicians and hospitals to in-network providers.
4. Use of out-of-network physicians and hospitals may result in huge out-of-pocket costs.
5. Many health plans refuse to pay for needed medical and surgical care.

Over the past 20 years the insurance industry has spent over $1 billion lobbying Congress, of which a large portion has come from health plans.

Campaign contributions to congressional candidates by the insurance industry exceeds $450 million, with estimates of nearly $200 million from health plans, over the past 20 years.

(In this chapter, health insurance companies are referred to as health plans interchangeably.)

My patients constantly complain to me about their health plans. On a single day in the winter of 2019, I listened to these:

"They lied. They don't cover the prescription drug that really helps me."

"I spend hours on the phone trying to find out why they refused to pay a portion of my hospital bill and only got handed off from one idiot to another idiot."

"What good is insurance when I pay the first $6,000 of outrageous costs out of my pocket?"

"How do I know which specialist is in-network and who is not? It seems to change every week."

These are only a few examples of the earful I hear from my patients. Every day I work in clinic I listen to complaints about health plans refusing to pay for medical care. Back in the days when I worked in the emergency department (ED), I heard horror stories of patients with painful and serious conditions that ended up in the ED because their health plans refused to allow them access to specialists and magnetic resonance imaging, or MRI. I would do the best I could to help them in the ED. Often health plans would refuse to pay for that ED visit, throwing my patients into bankruptcy.

In clinic, my medical assistant greets me each morning with a list of denials for care by health plans. A denial means that the health plan refuses to pay for important things the primary care doctor has ordered. This includes imaging (CT scans, MRIs, etc.), drugs, specialists' evaluations, hospitalizations, and surgery. I consider these denials to pay for health care like roadblocks on a highway.

Sometimes I can steer around a roadblock, and other times the health plan has cleverly figured out how to refuse care. At times, I can help the referral nurse navigate through a gauntlet of questions on a computer screen created by the health plan. Many of these "trick" questions have been framed in a way that will deliberately deny approval of a service or referral. Collectively, I have spent hours going through the appeal process with health plan administrative physicians. How can they deny care without ever examining my patient? Does the health plan appeals physician even have a medical license, and if so from where? Will these authorization physicians get a bonus or a promotion for denying care? My take-home impression after each day of clinical work of the for-profit insurance industry is *health plans deny needed and sometimes lifesaving medical care so the shareholders and CEO can pocket more of the health care premiums for themselves.* But they defend their actions by telling me they are not denying care; they are just refusing to pay.

Let's start this chapter with a list of the top 10 "money middlemen," corporations involved with health care insurance, using 2018 data:

1. United Healthcare Group, New York Stock Exchange (NYSE): UNH, 49 million members
2. Anthem, NYSE: ANTM, 40 million members
3. Aetna, NYSE: AET, 22 million members
4. Health Care Services Corp., customer owned: 15 million members
5. Cigna, NYSE: CI, 15 million members
6. Humana, NYSE: HUM, 14 million members
7. Centene Corporation, NYSE: CNC, 12 million members
8. Kaiser Permanente, nonprofit: 10.7 million members
9. WellCare Health Plans, NYSE: WCG, 6 million members
10. Highmark, nonprofit: 4.5 million members

Seven of these 10 corporations are for-profit, most paying dividends to shareholders and enormous salaries and bonuses to the bosses. *Modern Healthcare* published a list of CEO compensation for 2016, which included Centene's CEO, Michael Neidorff, who received $22 million. Is a for-profit system of health care insurance an essential component of health care delivery? No. Europe is an example in which most health plans are nonprofit or government run.

Some people think that because they have a health plan vetted by their employer it will be a good plan. One example is described in box 4.1: an "insured" patient with a $108,000 out-of-pocket bill for a $164,000 hospital charge. My patients also complain about being cheated by their employer-based health plans and having to pay out of pocket for imaging and procedures that I think are critical, yet the health plan refuses to pay.

The Evolution of Health Insurance Corporations and Health Maintenance Organizations

Health care insurance had its origins in nineteenth-century Europe. In the 1880s, Germany established an insurance program called Krankenversicherungsgesetz, a government-run program that required both

Kaiser Health News and NPR published a story in September 2018 describing a teacher who was hospitalized at St. David's Hospital in Texas. A high school history teacher in Austin, Texas, collapsed in his bedroom from a heart attack. A neighbor rushed him to the nearby emergency department at St. David's Medical Center on April 2, 2017. St. David's Healthcare, a large hospital system in central Texas, is operated by for-profit Hospital Corporation of America. The ED doctors diagnosed a heart attack and admitted him to the hospital's cardiac unit. The next day, doctors implanted stents in his clogged arteries. The hospital charged $164,941 for his surgery and four days in the hospital (see chapter 2, Hospitals, for real cost vs. profits). Aetna, which administers health benefits for the Austin Independent School District, paid the hospital $55,840. Who was on the hook for the unpaid portion of the bill, more than $100,000? The teacher. He had believed he would not pay much, if any, out-of-pocket cost, since he had a health plan. But since the health plan did not pay, the hospital then billed the teacher for the unpaid balance of $108,951.31. After national media coverage, the hospital reduced the teacher's out-of-pocket cost to $322. I encourage the reader of this book to read the many stories published by *Kaiser Health News* in its Bill of the Month section.

employers and employees to contribute to health care insurance that would cover the costs of illness of city workers. In the United States, the first insurance programs began in the 1920s as small nonprofit entities, offering to cover the cost of hospitalization for a low annual fee. By the 1940s, only about 2% of the US population had either hospital, doctor medical insurance, or both. At that time, most persons paid for medical care with cash or would be granted credit and make small payments over time. In rural areas, physicians would accept firewood, chickens, or a few hours of labor in exchange for medical care.

The health care landscape changed with World War II. Unionized workers could not strike for higher wages under the legal constraints of the war. Instead, they were granted a tax-free benefit of employer-paid health care insurance. For-profit insurance companies jumped into the business of health care. Employers of nonunionized workers also began offering insurance as a benefit. By 1960, nearly 70% of the US population had some form of health care insurance. In 1965, the federal Medicare program for persons aged 65 years and older provided coverage after workers retired. Health care insurance was affordable and, in many cases, 100% paid by the employer.

Medicine became more complex and expensive beginning in the early 1960s. New drugs and new procedures such as endoscopy, colonoscopy, arthroscopy, open-heart surgery, CT scans, intensive care units, and cancer treatments added to an accelerating cost of health care. Insurance paid. Hospitals and physicians learned they could inflate the bills of patients and send these outrageously high bills to health plans, further raising the costs for the health plans. A retired hospital executive once told me: "It was unbelievable. We could charge almost any amount and they would pay, why charge one cent for a Tylenol tablet, when they would pay us $20 for one pill!" I was actually interviewed on national television by ABC's Sam Donaldson on outrageous hospital charges. And, yes, I had to defend the hospital's $20 for a single Tylenol pill charge, which I regret now.

So health plans raised their rates and began refusing to pay the full amount of hospital charges and doctor fees. But insurance corporations also saw an opportunity to make more money by holding on to some of the billions of dollars flowing through their treasuries. That would make company executives and stockholders happy. And as long as they paid for most of the medical care, people would not care. But employers began to complain about the rising costs of insurance, and when they passed some of the costs onto employees, finally everyone started complaining. Then health plans began denying coverage for persons with preexisting conditions who were not covered by an employee health plan. Even more complaints from the public surfaced in the media.

To control costs and offer cheaper plans, some health plans began to create health maintenance organizations (HMOs). An HMO, generally speaking, is less expensive than a "full choice of any doctor" health plan. But HMOs limit medical care to a few predetermined hospitals and doctors and usually require approval by the HMO for referrals to specialists, surgical procedures, and drugs. I even wrote a peer-reviewed article in an emergency medicine scientific journal describing a practice of HMOs refusing to pay for ED visits when patients had true emergency medical conditions (Derlet 1997).

Unlike Kaiser, which is a closed system that combines the insurer and the provider, these new HMOs contracted with private physicians, paying them low rates but guaranteeing patient volume. In addition, HMOs negotiated rates with hospitals and severely restricted patient access to specialists, cancer treatments, surgical procedures, and other medical care. Dr. Linda Peeno, who worked as a medical reviewer for Humana, testified to the US Congress on the "dirty work" of HMOs. She gave as an example her denying lifesaving surgery to a patient and saving the company $500,000 (testimony to US Congress, May 30, 1996).

In 1992, Bill Clinton was elected president with a promise to fix the problem of rising health care costs and insurance coverage and HMO denials of medical care. He assigned Hillary Clinton to chair a task force on health care reform. The 1993 task force proposals, which included expansion of health coverage and benefits, was met with fierce opposition. Foremost among the opponents was the insurance industry, which faced losing billions in profits.

By defeating the Clinton health plan, insurance corporations had a green light to continue on the road to higher profits. Many nonprofit insurance executives saw an opportunity to get rich and converted nonprofit to for-profit corporations. Blue Cross's conversion to Anthem Blue Cross is an example of a health plan that became for-profit and is listed on the NYSE as ANTM. Its stock price increased from $30 a share to $289 a share from 2003 to 2019. That's corporate medicine. However, not all health plans are profit focused. Kaiser health plans deliver good care for a reasonable price. But many health plans continue to refuse to pay for needed care, as discussed at the beginning of this chapter. Another example is proved in box 4.2.

Definitions of Common Health Plan Terms

To understand the complexities of health insurance, it is important to understand a few commonly used terms. The dollar amounts are the ballpark ranges.

Box 4.2

The first example (box 4.1) of the teacher initially stuck with a $100,000 out-of-pocket bill may be legal because the hospital narrowly jumped through a legal loophole at the expense of the patient. Here is an example of insurance cheating that clearly violates health care law and regulations:

In March 2015, my 95-year-old father was returning from a supermarket with a grocery bag half filled with milk and bananas in Los Angeles, California. He had to cross a busy street on his way home. The signal light at the corner of Ambrose Avenue and Hillhurst Boulevard turned green, and the pedestrian crosswalk light glowed "walk" for him to cross the street. Suddenly, a car screeched around the corner and struck him, knocking him down onto the concrete of the four-lane boulevard. Someone called 9-1-1, and soon the Los Angeles Fire Department ambulance arrived. The paramedics discovered my father lying in the street covered with blood and nearly unconscious. As required by protocol, the paramedics rushed the "injured 95-year-old with altered mental status" to the Los Angeles County USC Emergency Trauma Center. He was hospitalized for five days.

My sister, Marian, who handled Dad's finances, soon received a bill for nearly $2,000 for the cost of the ambulance. She contacted the health plan, expecting them to pay everything, except the $100 deductible for ambulance service. The $100 maximum out of pocket for ambulance transport was actually printed on the back of his health care identification card. But the health plan refused to pay, stating that the ambulance transport was not preauthorized.

What? A 95-year-old man, run over by a car on a busy Los Angeles street, laying on the concrete had to call to get an ambulance authorized? Yes, in this case, and what a dirty trick to avoid paying the $2,000 ambulance charge.

Dad had assigned his Medicare benefit to a health plan as the Part C option Medicare beneficiaries have, called Medicare Care Advantage. Under this option, the government pays a fixed sum to the HMO or insurance company, who in return promises to provide medical care. How much the government pays varies by state, location, risk conditions, and so forth but is in the ballpark of $10,000 a year. We will discuss Medicare Part C later in this chapter.

The health plan received big bucks to care for my dad and then refused to pay when he needed to be rescued by the paramedics after being run over on a LA street. So after repeated threatening notices from the ambulance unit, and repeated calls to the health plan, my sister finally

Employer health care premium contribution. Money paid directly
from the employer (e.g., Stanford University) to the health plan. Range:
$8,000–$12,000 per year per employee. Double that amount (yes,
$24,000 per year) for a family plan.

Employee health care premium contribution. Money deducted from
employees' paychecks as their contribution to employer-sponsored
health care insurance. Range: $3,600–$4,800 per year for a single employee, and double or more for a family plan. I have seen family plan
employee contributions as high as $16,000 a year.

Co-pay. Out-of-pocket money paid for each doctor visit or prescription. Range: $10–$40.

Annual deductible. Out-of-pocket money a person must pay before
insurance starts to pay (exception: to see in-network physician, just
pay co-pay). Range: $1,500–$6,000 a year.

Co-insurance. This is a confusing term. It refers to the percentage
of the charge a person pays out of pocket after the deductible has been
reached. If a surgery bill is $10,000, and the insured's health plan has
a 25% co-insurance, the health plan would pay $7,500, and the in-
sured person would pay $2,500.

Annual out-of-pocket maximum. This rule was created to prevent
insured individuals from paying unlimited money on health care. Many
plans require a 20% contribution from the patient for a hospitalization, which can be huge if you are talking about 20% of a $300,000
hospital charge. So, when a person has paid a certain amount out of
pocket, the health plan pays every dollar beyond that. Out-of-pocket

expenses can be as low as $1,500 to as high as $8,000 per person (family plan range: $3,000–$16,000), above which insurance pays 100% for approved care. But there are many exclusions regarding what costs a health plan may actually pay.

Authorization for procedures, drugs, specialty visits, and surgery. Insurance may not pay for these unless they are approved in advance. If they are not approved, people may be stuck paying 100% of the bill. An unauthorized MRI may cost $8,000. A patient may be stuck with a bill that eventually may be sent to a collection agency.

In network versus out of network. In network means a doctor or a hospital has a contract with the insurance company, generally with a huge discount. Example: the hospital retail charge for a hip replacement is $120,000. The insurance company contracts in advance for $50,000. The insurance company pays some, and the insured person pays the rest to reach the $50,000. The patient cannot be "balance billed" for the additional $70,000. However, if the hospital is out of network, the full retail charge of $120,000 may be applied.

Health savings account (HSA). Money is set aside tax free matched by the employer and used to pay for health care. The amount of $3,500 a year is a drop in the ocean of costs. Initially the concept was to entice people to shop for the best deal. HSAs are discussed in a separate section in this chapter.

Medical loss ratio. The amount the insurance company spends on health care versus administration, profit, redundancy, and inefficiency. When dollars are spent on medical care, it is called a loss. The Affordable Care Act (ACA) requires health plans to spend 75%–80% on real health care.

Surprise medical bills. We touched on surprise doctor bills in chapter 3. The hospital component of a surprise medical bill hits patients even harder than the doctor side. Surprise bills occur when a patient goes to a hospital that is out of network. Since the insurance company does not have a contract with the hospital, the patient is billed at the highest retail rate; the insurance company may pay what it thinks is reasonable, which ballpark is 30%–50% of the retail rate. The hospital then demands that patients pay the difference, in a practice called *balance billing*. Several states have passed laws to help shield consumers from surprise bills and balance billing, particularly for emergency care. But there's a huge loophole, and some state-mandated protections may not apply to everyone, for example people who get their health coverage from employers that are self-insured. Several bills were introduced in the US Congress in 2019 that would end surprise medical bills. However no measure was approved, in part because of lobbying by Wall Street–type investor groups.

Provider. A clinical health care specialist, the term most commonly includes physicians, nurse practitioners, and physician assistants.

The Nuts and Bolts of the Current System

America has one of the most complex systems in the world to pay for health care services. This ranges from patients paying 100% cash for services to health plans that cover 100% of the cost for services. The methods by which health plans transfer money to doctors and hospitals are many, and I have described a few here.

The old traditional insurance type of payment system. The doctor/hospital bills the patient. The insured person (patient) submits their doctor/hospital/ancillary care bills to the insurance company and the patient is then reimbursed by receiving a check in the mail from the insurance company. Still used but uncommon.

Direct payment from insurance to doctors and hospitals. In this scheme, the hospitals and physicians directly bill the insurance company. The insurance company then pays 80%–100% of the fee. The insurance company sends no money to the patient. The insurance may require that the patient pay a percentage of the charge and require prior authorization for some imaging, procedures, and surgeries.

Limited direct payment from health plan to contracted doctors and hospitals. Commonly used with preferred provider organization (PPO) systems: The hospital and physician directly bill the insurance company. The insurance company pays the hospital and physician at a pre-negotiated rate, usually 50%–80% of the retail fee. No money is sent to the patient. But patients must use in-network-assigned doctors and hospitals. The patient is responsible for the portion of the bill not paid by the insurance entity but at the contracted rate. The hospital retail rate for a hip replacement is $100,000. The insurance company has negotiated a contracted rate of $60,000. The insurance pays $48,000 (80% of $60,000) leaving the patient with $12,000 to pay out of pocket. At an out-of-network hospital, the patient may be responsible for $62,000 ($100,000 – $48,000) or, in some cases, the full $100,000 fee.

Some HMOs use contracted doctors and hospitals. This health plan is responsible for delivering all medical care to the enrolled person and enrolled family members. Generally, this means the health plan contracts with specific hospitals and doctors who must take care of the person. The insured person must go to these in-network facilities or they will have to pay some or the entire bill. If a person requires emergency treatment in an ED, HMO plans may provide an exception for care in out-of-network hospitals and pay for all or a portion of the care.

Fully independent-standing HMO. This health plan owns and operates hospitals and clinics and employs physicians. The best-known system is Kaiser Permanente Healthcare. A person who signs up agrees to only use facilities owned or approved by the HMO.

Common Types of US Health Plans
Employer Health Plans

Employer-sponsored health insurance still dominates the landscape. About 50% of the population has these health plans. The employer shops around, considering one or more insurance plans, to cover its employees. The employer (for example, the XYZ Company) negotiates the actual benefits to match what both XYZ and the worker will pay. In the past, before the recent rise in health care costs, XYZ might pay 90%. So, if a total cost of insurance was $400 a month, XYZ would deduct $40 a month from the employee paycheck and pay that and the balance of $360 to the insurance company.

The cost of providing insurance has skyrocketed. Now a plan might cost as much as $12,000 a year for a single employee and $24,000 a year for a family plan. The employee increasingly picks up more of the cost, in some cases seeing paycheck deductions of as much as $500 a month. A benefit of employer-sponsored plans: insurance coverage cannot be refused because of preexisting conditions.

What benefits does a person receive? Doctor visits are covered after a co-pay of $20–$50 each visit, provided a person sees a physician in network, a physician with a contract with the health plan. Certain drugs are covered with a co-pay. For other expenses, the individual pays out of pocket until the deductible is reached, and that may range from $1,000 to $6,000. Thereafter, the insurance pays between 60% and 80% until the person reaches the out-of-pocket annual maximum, usually $12,000. In theory, the health plan pays everything thereafter, but a dizzying number of exceptions may exist. Similar to the in-network physicians' restriction, the same applies to hospitals: go to an out-of-network hospital and you may have little if any paid by the health plan.

The enormous cost of health care insurance to employers is an important issue but has not received its fair share of attention and discussion in the national media. For example, GM pays $4.5 billion annually for health care insurance, adding $1,200 to the cost of each vehicle manufactured. In some respects, the high cost of "corporate medicine" is driving American corporations to move factories overseas.

Health Savings Accounts

Employers can also offer an HSA in conjunction with a high-deductible employee health plan. The employee can elect to transfer up to $3,500 a year of earnings into a special tax-free account for medical expenses. The intent of the law that created the HSA was to stimulate free market "shopping," drive down medical costs, and lower some out-of-pocket expenses. But this does not work when prices are not posted, and getting a hospital or clinic to divulge its prices is nearly impossible. Similar programs include medical savings accounts and flexible spending accounts. These all have rules too complex for me to understand. My patients who have tried one of these systems often find out-of-pocket expenses actually increase, and they opt back into a traditional health plan during the next open enrollment.

Health Plans Purchased on the Open Market

In this model, individuals purchase insurance on their own accord. This group constitutes 10% of the population. Who are these people? They include the self-employed, unemployed, contract workers, some part-time workers, and employees whose employers do not provide health insurance. By current law, employers with more than 50 workers are required to provide health care insurance.

Before enactment of the ACA in 2010, insurance companies could exclude persons with preexisting conditions. An insurer could retrospectively cancel a policy after a major medical expense. For example, if a person forgot to list on their application for health insurance that they were treated for acne as a teenager, they would be accused of falsifying their application, and faced cancellation of the policy, leaving them on the hook for a giant medical bill.

Purchasing health insurance on your own can be a prohibitive cost. Who has $24,000 in loose change to buy a family plan? The ACA addressed one element of cost. States were provided with federal funds and a structure to establish their own insurance exchanges. In California, the exchange is known as Covered California. In states that refuse to participate, individuals could get insurance through a federal exchange program. A sliding scale was used to determine what an individual would pay for insurance. Federal and state contributions are as much as 90% for those in the lower-income brackets. Government contributions phase out once family income is above $90,000. In addition, the ACA guaranteed funding directly to certain health plans if they incurred a loss from the new program.

The standardized plans come in four categories: Bronze, Silver, Gold, and Platinum. The plans that provide more comprehensive insurance are more expensive. Many people complain about the Bronze level insurance. It carries a deductible of over $6,000 a person a year or $12,000 for the family plan. Until a person has forked out-of-pocket their $6,000 deductible, the health plan may not pay for any medical expenses except for a few doctor visits, and even then, with co-pays as much as $90. One of my patients said to me: "It's like having no insurance; almost every charge is for me to pay." This lower tier was intended to be catastrophic, to save having an auto or home repossessed. So many people do not own a home, and their auto is "owned" by a lending bank that gave them an auto loan. But Bronze is all some families can afford.

Medicare

Medicare is one of the best-known health care insurance programs, covering 15% of the population, and proposed by many members of Congress as a model for all Americans. Medicare was one of President Lyndon Johnson's Great Society initiatives and took effect in 1965. To be eligible for Medicare a person must be age 65 or older and have 40 quarters, or 10 years, of paying Social Security/Medicare payroll taxes.

The benefits of Medicare include the following:

- Part A: covers inpatient hospitalization and is free care minus a deductible, which is currently $1,408.
- Part B: covers non-inpatient care and costs $145 a month (in 2020) for married couples earning less than $170,000 a year (90% of recipients). Part B pays for 80% of charges.
- Part C: also called Medicare Advantage. This is an HMO option.
- Part D: prescription benefit. Enacted in 2003, the purpose of Part D is to provide some federal funding for prescription drugs, thus reducing out-of-pocket costs for a beneficiary.
- Nearly all hospitals and most physicians accept Medicare.
- Medicare sets the maximum fee it will pay for services for those in Parts A and B. In most cases, this is 30%–50% of the "retail" charge listed. Most important, people cannot be billed the difference of the retail charge (balanced billing).

The problems with traditional Medicare include the following:

- Part B only covers 80% of the Medicare set fee. When the law was adapted in 1965, Part B paid for physicians' fees as well as outpatient simple lab tests and x-rays. Many times these were done in the physician's office. It does not cover ED charges, and in the 1960s not much was done in the ED compared to the present. If someone was sick or injured, they would be admitted, with costs covered by Part A. Now, an ED evaluation can cost $20,000; the 20% not covered by Medicare Part B is $4,000. Many people buy "gap" insurance to cover this portion of expenses not covered by Medicare. If secondary insurance is not part of an employer retirement benefit, purchasing gap insurance can be expensive, about $300 a month.
- Physicians may up-code the level of the visit to claim a higher dollar fee. To prevent this, Medicare is in the process of developing a one universal fee for an office visit.
- The Medicare Modernization Act of 2003 Part D, a drug payment for Medicare. The law prohibits Medicare from negotiating prices for drugs, and the Part D is subcontracted to corporate entities, basically privatizing the program. Big Pharma is making a fortune by inflating the "list price" of a drug minus a small discount. And, in an unusual quirk, not all drugs are covered. I have patients paying more than $100 a month or more out of pocket for a single drug. This is a problem when a retiree survives on $1,000 a month from Social Security. So some of my retired patients on Social Security and Medicare go to church-sponsored food banks to eat.

Medicare Advantage Plan. The intent of the Medicare Advantage Plan is threefold: (1) to reduce overall out-of-pocket costs to seniors, (2) to offer additional benefits not provided by traditional Medicare, and (3) to have the assigned health plan manage overall health expenditures. Nearly a third of Medicare recipients have assigned their benefits to a private corporate health plan. In this model, the federal government pays a health plan a fixed amount per year, in the ballpark of

$10,000 per year per person. The health plan is responsible for providing all medical care. In some areas of the country, this works well. The Kaiser health system receives high marks for care to those persons over age 65.

But Medicare Advantage restricts the choice of doctors and hospitals a person may choose. In some cases, doctors listed as in network are located far away, are not accepting new patients, or do not interact well with elderly people. The corporate health plan may deny or limit care as described at the beginning of this chapter (see box 4.2), when the health plan refused to pay for the $2,000 ambulance cost for a 95-year-old man run over by a car in Los Angeles. Wrong hospital? Wrong doctor? The senior pays.

In late 2019, I called several health plans offering the Medicare Advantage Plan. My question: What if a person was taken to an out-of-network hospital ED, for what they perceived as an emergency medical condition, but retroactively the health plan determined it was not an emergency? I could not get a clear answer. But judging from actions of the past by health plans, I worry that they could refuse to pay the bill, leaving the senior on the hook to pay the hospital ED charge in full, which could cost in the tens of thousands of dollars.

Other means of cheating has been described for corporate health plans receiving Medicare Advantage funding. Some may attempt to get more money from the government by falsely up-coding. A provision allows for higher annual payments to HMOs that care for high-risk people. Health plans have been accused of placing people in a high-risk category when in fact they are not high risk.

Medicaid

Medicaid began with the passage of the Social Security Amendments of 1965 and covers 20% of the population. The program provided states with the framework for assisting vulnerable populations' access to medical care. In California, Medicaid is known as Medi-Cal. Although the program is managed by individual states, the federal government provides states 50% of the program cost and sets many of the rules and regulations. Initially, the largest eligible populations were children from low-income single parents. The 2010 ACA expanded eligibility requirements to include nearly anyone who fell below certain poverty-line income definitions.

The benefits of Medicaid include the following:

- It's free; recipients pay no cost or co-pays.
- There is no balanced billing. Hospitals and doctors cannot bill a patient for the difference between what Medicaid pays and the retail rate.
- Nearly all non-psychiatric hospitals accept Medicaid.

The problems with Medicaid include the following:

- Since payments to doctors are lower than Medicare in many states, the selection of physicians may be limited. In some locations, the only option for care is to use a hospital emergency department.
- Some states have contracted with Wall Street corporations to manage their Medicaid programs. These corporations may severely limit access to imaging, drugs, and specialists.

HMOs That Own Their Health Care Facilities

You might be asking, weren't HMOs covered in the "employer sponsored section"? Yes, employers can buy Kaiser for employees in some locations, but this model deserves special mention. In this model, the HMO acts both as an insurance company and as a health delivery organization. Kaiser owns its hospitals and employs the doctors, pharmacists, nurses, and ancillary staff needed to provide the full spectrum of health care. It is a leader in attempting to find the best path for cost-effective health care. It is truly a closed system, limiting individuals to only Kaiser facilities. But they are very good at transferring their patients out of non-Kaiser EDs should someone go there in an emergency.

Health Plans and the High Cost of Medical Care

Health plans have attempted to put the brakes on the runaway train of outrageous health care costs. They fight monopoly practices of hospitals, physicians, and Big Pharma. They negotiate with hospitals to set prices less than the hospital retail rate. As a generalization, think about 50% of the retail rate of a hospital bill. But it may be difficult to negotiate with hospitals that have regional monopolies—that is, no other hospital within 100 or more miles—demand more, as well as academic centers which may demand a contract that pays as much as 80% of retail. For physicians, health plans try to negotiate the Medicare rate, about $100 for the most common median-level visit.

Methods Health Plans May Use to Mislead, Fool, Cheat, or Trick

Some people feel tricked when they learn that their health plan refuses to pay for certain health care costs, fees, and bills. As I noted in the beginning of the chapter, my patients have used the following words in relating their health plan experiences: *confusing, cheating, swindlers, con artists, tricked, lying, deceptive, misleading, racket, scam,* and many others. I will refer to the practices that follow as tricks.

Trick 1: Limited or no choice of hospitals or doctors. A person signs up with a health care plan and feels happy and secure. Then they learn they can only see physicians who are on the official list of in-network physicians. These physicians may be miles away from their homes. In addition, physicians on the list may not be accepting new patients, forcing people to drive even farther to find an available physician. It may be even worse to see specialists. I once had a patient who needed an evaluation from an ear, nose, and throat specialist. The only ENT was 200 miles away. The patient did not have a car. He got a neighbor to make the five-hour drive, only to find the appointment cancelled.

In addition, people must use in-network hospitals. Going to the wrong hospital may result in the health plan refusing to pay or, in the best circumstances, paying at a low rate, say, 40% of the retail charge.

At out-of-network hospitals, a person may be on the hook for balanced billing. If the retail rate were $100,000, and the insurance paid $40,000, the patient would owe $60,000. Hospitals are notorious for sending unpaid bills to collection agencies. And don't forget about drugs. A person may not have drugs covered if they go to an out-of-network pharmacy or have a prescription for an unapproved drug.

Trick 2: Refusing to pay for items legally mandated by contract or law. The first example (box 4.1) of the teacher stuck with a $100,000 out-of-pocket bill narrowly jumped through a legal loophole at the expense of the patient. In another case, an HMO plan refused to pay for emergency care for a man after being struck by a vehicle on a busy Los Angeles street (box 4.2). One of my patients was stuck with a bill for emergency care after her health plan refused to consider severe pain an emergency (box 4.3).

Trick 3: Roadblocks and detours in approving procedures and specialists. Need a referral to a specialist, an MRI, or hernia surgery? Your health plan may require *prior authorization*. Prior authorization means the physician's office must explain why a person needs the referral for

---

Box 4.3

A 48-year-old female patient of mine awoke at 2 a.m. with severe back pain and confusion. Her husband did the commonsense thing and drove her to a nearby emergency department. An evaluation in the ED showed she had dangerously high blood pressure and left kidney infection, which required immediate administration of antibiotics. Her health plan refused to pay her $6,600 ED bill, stating that she did not have an emergency. This flies in the face of federal law, which defines "severe pain" as an emergency medical condition. She had severe pain, as well as symptoms that mimicked a stroke (confusion). One of the reasons we pay for health care insurance is to cover unexpected emergencies.

I am not the only front line physician who has seen up-front health plans refusing to pay for ED care. A *Consumer Reports* article described how Anthem was accused of 1,600 payment denials for ED care (Rosato 2018). Some members of Congress are aware of the "refusing to pay for ED care" problem but have failed to act. More related ED issues are discussed in chapter 7.

anything from MRI imaging to surgery. The health plan may require a phone call or going through a computer algorithm.

Each day in my primary care I encounter patients who are denied authorization for care, procedures, or imaging by health plans. This is practicing medicine without examining the patient. One case that comes to mind is the patient who hobbled down the office hallway on crutches with great difficulty and in severe pain. The pain was so severe that our staff could see the agony in her sweat-dripping face. She had a ruptured spinal disc and had been denied an MRI of the lumbar-sacral spine by her health plan, a study I needed to get her referred to a spine surgeon. It is not right for a person hundreds or even thousands of miles away to have the power to deny proper care. Health plans use authorization denials to save money. Patients are left in pain and suffering. Yes, we can appeal, but this takes mountains of time, hassles, and frustration. I have waited on the phone for over 30 minutes to speak to a health plan physician to get an authorization.

Trick 4: Claiming physicians are available, when they are not. A long list of in-network physicians may be provided at open enrollment, but only a few physicians may be accepting patients.

Trick 5: Limiting and overcharging prescription drugs. Health plans may not cover some vital prescription drugs. Health plans have various tiers of drugs on their approved list called *formularies.* I saw a corporate formulary that was only two pages. Normally, they should be hundreds of pages. In theory, the physician can appeal to have a nonformulary drug covered. However, contacting a health plan, in order to get a nonformulary drug approved can take 15 or 20 minutes of time, and result in a backup of patients waiting to be seen in a busy clinic. And the end result may be that the requested nonformulary drug is not approved.

A recent study found that 25% of the time people pay more of a co-pay for a prescription drug than the actual cost of the drug (Van Nuys 2018). In one case cited in the media, a person paid a $240 co-pay for a drug costing $40 retail (Thompson 2018). In another example, the same report describes a co-pay through insurance of $120 for a drug with a retail cost of $35.

Trick 6: Selling junk insurance. Not all health plans are the same. The ACA attempted to standardize many of the important benefits provided by health plans while still allowing some differences and consumer choice (see chapter 9). It abolished junk insurance. Prior to the ACA, junk insurance that was sold might cover only the first $3,000 to $5,000 of medical bills, limit paid doctor visits, or pay a small fraction of the cost of hospitalization. These plans limited services covered such as maternity care. The federal government issued a new rule in 2018 that again allowed junk insurance. In October 2018, Congress attempted to overturn the rule, but failed.

Trick 7: Not telling patients about balanced billing. Suppose you go to an in-network hospital and have surgery by an in-network surgeon and think, because of insurance company contracts, you are responsible for a fraction of the bill. After all the health plan has a contract with the hospital and doctor, right? Wrong. You will be stuck paying your deductible (up to $6,500) and out-of-pocket fractions up to the maximum annual out-of-pocket level (up to $13,000). You may not be done with out-of-pocket expenses once you reach $13,000. If the ancillary physicians and lab were out of network, you will receive a bill for those services. Also referred to as "surprise medical bills," balanced billing is an out-of-pocket expense to pay the difference between what the insurance pays, and the full retail charge. For example, an out-of-network anesthesiologist bills the insurance company $5,000 of which your insurance pays $1,000. You will still owe $4,000, the balanced bill. The term "balanced billing" usually refers to a full retail charge, and not a contracted charge negotiated between a health plan and hospital or doctor. Why were you not told this in advance?

Trick 8: Claiming mergers will improve care. We read frequently about large Wall Street mergers, buyouts, or other tricks to combine two or three companies into one big monopoly. These big mergers, involving banks, telecommunications companies, airlines, and oil corporations, have become common: more monopoly power means more profit. The health care industry in many aspects has become a for-profit industry, placing profits ahead of patient welfare. For-profit insurance corporations that have merged include Aetna and Humana and Anthem and Cigna. As with other Wall Street mergers, monopolies increase cost and limit choice.

Trick 9: Delaying payments to providers for care. My office biller has repeatedly sent me notifications via the computer to go into a patient's electronic medical record to add additional information to the EMR to one of my office visits of that patient. For example, ask about a history of smoking. Failure to provide this information may result in the health plan not paying for the person's visit. This is basically a stall tactic, for the health plan to get out of paying. For example a health plan may refuse to pay for an office visit for a patient with poison oak, because I did not ask about a history of alcohol intake. I spoke with the office manager of a small surgical practice who told me it was routine for health plans to refuse to pay for a person's surgery when the bill was initially submitted and that a bill might have to be sent multiple times to be paid. The *Modesto Bee* described how a health plan that insured city employees refused to pay $8 million in claims, resulting in some patients' bills being sent to collection agencies (Valine 2019).

Trick 10: Hiding behind civil law. Health plans that cheat people usually face no consequences. A person's only recourse may be to hire an attorney. But paying a $5,000 attorney retainer fee to fight a $4,000 "refusal to pay a medical bill" is a barrier most people cannot afford. There is no police force to throw lawbreaking health plans in jail (or their CEOs). Many health care laws are governed under civil law, meaning if a person is wronged, that person will need to hire an attorney to take cheaters to court. Why has not Congress made more of the regulations to be criminal law with fines and jail time? Some experts in health care law argue we need a regulatory agency to protect consumers, similar to the Consumer Finance Protection Bureau.

Actions to Protect People and Decrease Health Plan Charges

Outlaw campaign contributions and lobbying to Congress by the health plan industry. Contributions to election campaigns for Congress come with a string—the members of Congress get money for their campaigns and then are expected to support legislation favorable to the health insurance industry. How can a US senator or representative vote in the best interest of the people when future contributions to their political campaigns depend on their voting in favor of corporate profits. Take a look at some of the big bucks that members of Congress have received: Huge contributions by the health insurance industry influenced the ACA. For example, they "vetoed" the public option.

Blue Cross Blue Shield spent $23.8 million on lobbying to Congress and gave $5,385,000 in cash to political campaigns in 2018. Cigna spent $7.4 million on lobbying and over $1 million in campaign contributions. In all, over 80 of 100 US senators have received campaign contributions from health care insurance corporations. Will they vote in the best interest of the corporation or in the best interest of the average American?

Place real limits on the dollars the industry retains for profit and administration. Most European countries limit the amount of money a health plan can retain to 3%–5% of premiums collected. Can this be done in the United States? Absolutely. Medicare does it, retaining 3%–5% for administrative costs. European nonprofit insurance companies also have minimal administrative fees. The ACA limits should be revised to be consistent with European health plans.

Reduce high deductibles. No one should have to pay an annual $8,000 deductible. Deductibles of $500 to $1,000 a year would be more in line with European systems.

End the in-network, out-of-network game. Standardize payment for charges like Medicare at all physicians and hospitals.

End balanced billing. Prohibit balanced billing to the patient in disputes between the health plan and the entity that delivers health care.

Set limits on denial of covered services. Yes, it may be reasonable to refuse in advance to pay for certain cosmetic procedures and other purely elective medical care. But denial of payment for cancer care, referral to specialists, and imaging and procedures deemed necessary by the primary care physician should be prohibited.

Reclassify certain serious violations of health care laws and regulations from civil to criminal law. Administrators whose actions result in harm to patients should be subject to criminal court proceedings and face monetary fines and jail time.

Bottom line: Too many health plans make money by fooling, tricking, or outright cheating people. Congress needs to step up to the plate and enact legislation to protect people, instead of protecting the profits of health care corporations.

FIVE

European Systems of Health Care Delivery

KEY CONCEPTS

1. Citizens cannot be denied care for preexisting conditions.
2. Annual individual out-of-pocket expenses are small compared to the United States.
3. Excellent quality of health care at half the US cost.
4. Government agencies set prices.

Campaign contributions: Chapters in this book list major contributions that influence the US Congress. In Europe, each of the many countries has different rules governing campaign contributions for candidates and elected members of government. Contribution limits are strict, and a fraction of US campaign contributions. As a result campaign donations have less influence on health care policy and law compared to America.

Each time I step off an aircraft in Europe, I breathe a sigh of relief. If some medical catastrophe happens to me I will not be out hundreds of thousands of dollars for out-of-pocket medical care. Even if I am given a full bill for medical services, like a broken arm or sprained ankle, my "foreign-visitor price" will be a fraction of that charged in the United States, in some cases only 10% of the US retail price.

Many experts on health care policy look to Western Europe for solutions to our high cost of medical care. On average, health care costs are half the costs in America. This means roughly $6,000 per person per year is spent providing health care versus $12,000 or more in America (table 5.1). Most important, the quality of health care and outcome is equal to or better than the United States. This chapter explains their different systems and costs. Although I use the more generic term *Europe*, I am referring to Western Europe.

Not all European heath care systems are the same. Most countries developed different types of "universal health care" after World War II.

As countries emerged from the destruction and ruin of the war, governments decided to provide citizens health care as a human right. The average person was broke in the postwar years, and if he were lucky enough to be employed, wages were meager and he lived paycheck to paycheck. Health care was unaffordable as an out-of-pocket expense. Each country then adopted its own unique type of national health care.

Visiting tourists may have to pay the real cost of care. What if you get sick or injured while on vacation in Europe and your insurance back home in the United States refuses to pay? The good news is you will probably not end up homeless, living under a bridge. Persons who are not European Union citizens are billed the real cost of care, not the outrageous, high-profit retail rate charged in the United States.

Richard Good, a friend of mine, works as a backcountry wilderness ranger. He is tough as nails, but on a tightly packed flight to Europe, he developed a bad cough, and after several days of sightseeing in Ireland, he came down with a rip-roaring pneumonia. He was hospitalized in Belfast for four days. He received treatment for the lung infection and was billed $2,300. The retail price tag for treating that same pneumonia in some US hospitals approaches $40,000. Was his US health plan happy with his inexpensive care and savings of $37,000? No. The insurer balked at paying the $2,300, even though its brochure advertised medical care coverage overseas.

Charles Remington, another colleague of mine, and a professor at the University of California, Davis, developed severe abdominal pain after eating a five-course dinner in Southern France. His bill to consult a local specialist in gastroenterology, including an abdominal ultrasound, was $50. The medication that cured his ailment cost $5 at the local pharmacy. In the United States, a visit for abdominal pain at an emergency department can cost $20,000. I know, I'm an ED doctor and have seen these $20,000 hospital bills. You might think that you cannot compare an ED visit to an office visit. Unlike France, in the United States, it is rare to be seen in a private physician's office after hours. The on-call physician, when telephoned, will send a patient with severe abdominal pain to the ED.

While I was in Finland, I asked the hospital director of a major university hospital in Kuopio what a hospital actually charges a citizen's municipality (county of residence) to perform a hip replacement. The answer: about $8,000. Plus the hospital collects another $150 in out-of-pocket co-pays from the patient. That's all the hospital gets for performing the surgery for a hip replacement. And that $8,150 (calculated from euros) has to balance the books, pay the employees, buy supplies, and medications. Compare that to a $100,000 price tag for the same procedure in a California hospital. And I reviewed several bills for hip replacements that were slightly over $100,000!

Although each country has a different approach to universal health care, there are similarities:

1. Their structures depend on primary care physicians (PCPs) as the cornerstone for their entire health care system. The European equivalent of US PCPs are called general practitioners, or GPs. Similar to their US counterparts, the collective goal of GPs is to keep people healthy and out of the hospital. Unlike the American PCPs, a higher proportion of the European population has GPs, and besides keeping people healthy and out of the hospital, they also help keep costs low. This is one reason why Europe gets more bang for its health care buck.

2. All countries provide or require universal health care for their citizens. No one is excluded for preexisting conditions.

3. Government regulates the health care insurance industry much more tightly than the United States. Insurance companies can retain only 3%–5% of revenue for profit and overhead, compared to 20%–25% in the United States.

4. The government sets the maximum prices that physicians and hospitals can charge. Prices are set for most prescription medications. Diagnostic related group (DRG) methods are used to regulate hospital and clinic charges. A DRG is a bundled charge based on the patient's diagnosis. A hospital will receive one set fee for taking care of a patient with pneumonia. In contrast, if a US hospital cares for a pneumonia patient, the hospital will add up hundreds of charges for each item (e.g., a bandage) or service (e.g., blood draw), with profit margins

Table 5.1. Health care expenditures
by country (2018–)

Finland	$4,228
Great Britain	$4,070
France	$4,965
Germany	$5,986
Netherlands	$5,288
United States	$10,586[a]

Source: From Organisation for Economic
Co-operation and Development.
Note: Annual per person per year, averaged.
[a]Estimated at $12,000 for 2020.

on each item, resulting in enormous charges and profits. The exception is Medicare's DRG system.

5. Limited annual out-of-pocket charges can range from near zero in England to $800 in Finland. US out-of-pocket expenses may exceed $20,000, even with "comprehensive" health care insurance.

6. Optional private hospitals and physicians are allowed in most countries. The numbers of these "boutique hospitals" are small and only for those people willing to pay the extra cost or for those who have purchased optional private insurance.

Types of Health Care Systems in Europe

1. *Full ownership by the national government.* The National Health Service (NHS) in Great Britain is the best-known government-owned system. Doctors are employed by the national government or under government contract. Hospitals are owned and operated by the national government. Funding is provided as a portion of the national government tax revenue (e.g., United Kingdom, Ireland).

2. *Government ownership but decentralized control to municipalities.* In a decentralized system, doctors are employed or contracted by the local governments (e.g., Finland) or work on a capitated basis (e.g., Italy). Local governments operate hospitals and medical facilities. Funding is provided as a portion of the national government and local tax revenues (e.g., Spain, Italy). In some cases, this is

not a lump sum (e.g., Finland). Hospitals must support their entire operation on the bills they submit to the patient's local municipal government.

3. *Multipayer system with mixed public/private hospitals and physicians, and multiple private insurance companies.* Confusing arrays of schemes exist in many European countries—for example France, Germany, Holland, and others. In Holland, both private nonprofit and for-profit entities provide health care insurance coverage. In France, the government-run insurance program reimburses people 70%–80% of costs, with private insurance providing much of the balance from private funds. In Germany, patients have a small co-pay, usually about $10, for physician visits, but the majority of health care costs are covered by the government-run *sickness fund*, or SF. Revenue to pay for health care can come from a variety of sources, including the general tax fund and special payroll taxes paid for by the employee and employer. In addition, insurance companies receive funding from both government and patient payments.

Health Care Snapshot of Five Selected European Countries
Great Britain

As I have observed as a visiting professor, emergency departments and hospitals in Great Britain are equal to or exceed the quality of care delivered in the United States. Even in my US practice, I read and refer to British medical journal articles because the British are international leaders in defining the quality of medical care. The NHS provides care to all residents with a system of government-owned hospitals and contracted or employed physicians.

History. Prior to World War II, people paid fees for services at individualized doctors' offices where they obtained their medical care. Public hospitals were available for those with no money. After World War II, few people had the resources to pay for medical care. Recognizing this problem, the government established the NHS in 1948 with the goal of providing health care to everyone. It was funded by general tax revenue and has successfully provided care to over 95% of British citizens for the past 70 years.

Prices for medical care. Since there are no charges for most medical services, there is no need to set prices. There are exceptions, for example, prescription drugs cost £7 ($11) a prescription, which can be waived in some circumstances.

Insurance. Every citizen and legal resident is entitled to health care in the NHS without buying insurance. However, people can buy private insurance to receive care in private hospitals, but this optional insurance is selected by less than 10% of the population. In this subset of private insurance patients, about a third pay out of pocket for the insurance, and about two-thirds have private insurance as a benefit through an employer. Optional insurance does not cover NHS GP visits, just visits to specialists and private hospitals.

Maximum out-of-pocket cost per person per year. These costs can be zero, since health care is free, except for prescription drugs. Usually, out-of-pocket costs are less than $100 a year.

Access to care. Access to medical care is very good and can be through a scheduled GP appointment or in urgent situations through the emergency department.

- GPs: Eighty percent are seen in one to five days.
- Specialists: Most people with common outpatient problems are seen in two to six weeks, depending on urgency of referral.
- Emergency care: British EDs are called accident and emergency departments, referred to as A&E. Persons with emergencies can go to the A&E for immediate care, but, similar to the US waiting room, times have been a problem for less urgent problems.

Hospitals. There is no charge for care in NHS hospitals. Acutely ill or injured patients get immediate hospitalization. Wait times for nonurgent and elective surgery have been the focus of disapproval by those critical of the British system. But my experience with British wait times differ little compared to America, as many US health plans throw up roadblocks, detours, or flat-out refusals for nonurgent surgery, resulting in waits of weeks to months.

France

French hospitals are similar in quality to US hospitals and range from crowded and unkempt to ultra clean and uncrowded. But in all my visits to hospitals in France, one thing is nearly identical: the physicians provide the same excellent care and have the same support systems to provide medical care—CT scans, MRIs, and advanced surgical techniques.

History. Beginning in 1928, very basic health care insurance was provided to selected industrial workers. After World War II, national health care insurance was rolled out to the entire population.

Prices for medical care. Prices are set for medical care services. Rates are determined by negotiations among physicians, hospitals, government, insurers, employers, and other groups. Examples of fixed prices include $30 for a GP visit and $40–$50 for a specialist.

Insurance. All residents are required to have insurance through non-profit, government-regulated insurance providers (NHI). A payroll tax at the level of the worker's employer pays for 50% of the program. The remainder of the money comes from national tax revenues. NHI pays 70% of physicians' visits and 80% of hospital stays. People can purchase optional insurance to cover the portion (20%–30%) not paid for by the NHI. Employers also may provide optional insurance. Full optional insurance can be purchased for persons wishing to use fully private physicians and hospitals.

Maximum out-of-pocket cost per person per year. Maximum out-of-pocket cost per year depends on the type and severity of illness. In some cases, severe problems are 100% covered by insurance. As a rule of thumb, the maximum out-of-pocket sum paid by French residents is about $120 a year. A French resident's co-pay for a physician visit is 1 euro (1 euro = $1.11 as of January 2020).

Access to care. Access to care is similar to other European countries by directly contacting the GP's office or going directly to an ED:

- GPs: Appointments are generally within a week and can be the same day for urgent problems.
- Specialists: Access times are days to weeks, which is similar to the United States and depends on the severity of the problem.
- Emergency care: France has a world-famous public system called SAMU. A person calls 112 (the old number 1–5) to access trained medical personnel that provide medical advice. In urgent and emergent situations, an ambulance is dispatched and may have a young physician on board. Emergency departments provide advanced medical and trauma care and admit persons to the hospital similar to the United States.

Hospitals. Admissions come from the ED or are admitted directly by physicians. The government uses a DRG system to set hospital rates. DRG means the hospital is paid by diagnosis, not by number of bandages used or laboratory tests done. NHI and private co-insurance pays for nearly 100% of charges, meaning individual out-of-pocket costs are minimal.

Germany

German medical care is excellent. While I was serving as a visiting professor, in Leipzig, I was impressed by the knowledge and critical thinking of the young physicians that I interacted with in the hospitals.

History. Germany is known for providing the first required health care insurance for certain city workers beginning in the 1880s. Following World War II and the rebuilding during the Marshall Plan, a multitiered insurance system evolved.

Prices for medical care. Government-organized commissions of medical stakeholders set prices. Price-setting commissions are found at both the national and local level. Prices are regulated for physicians, hospital care, and prescription drugs.

Insurance. All persons with income less than 52,000 euros (EU), about $59,000, are required to sign up with a health plan called sickness fund, or SF, and can choose one from over 90 nonprofit insurers.

SFs are paid from a payroll tax of 7.5% for both the employee and the employer (total 15%) on the first 52,000 EU of income. Persons earning more than 52,000 EU may elect to opt out of the SF and then buy private insurance, which provides more choices of hospitals and doctors. There are two types of optional insurance, but both have regulated prices. The first is supplemental, for those in the SF program that covers a few services not covered by the SF, such as dental and eyeglasses. The second is full coverage, which can be purchased by high earners opting out of SFs. The cost varies by risk pool: young single persons have low costs, whereas middle-aged persons with families may pay as much as $10,000. Private insurers may charge more for preexisting conditions.

Maximum out-of-pocket cost per person per year. Co-pays for physician visits are in the $5–$10 range. Typical maximum out of pocket (beyond payroll tax) is less than $100 a year for those insured through the Sickness Fund.

Access to care. People can access medical care through a variety of options in Germany.

- GPs: Appointments within one day to one week.
- Specialists: Patients are seen the same day up to several weeks, depending on urgency.
- Emergency care: Germany has a highly advanced emergency medical service, or EMS. Persons with emergent problems call 112 to activate the EMS system. Ambulances are dispatched through regional systems and may include a physician for critical problems. Patients with traumatic injuries are transported to trauma centers. The physician specialty of emergency medicine has only recently evolved, and larger hospitals may internally triage patients to subsections of the ED staffed by specialists in internal medicine, obstetrics and gynecology, pediatrics, and others.

Hospitals. German hospitals can be owned and operated by one of many entities, including local and regional governments (50%), nonprofit groups (35%), and private companies (15%). Admission to the hospital occurs through EDs or specialists.

Netherlands

I love visiting Holland and enjoy the diversity of the country, from bustling Amsterdam to international-flavored Den Haag (The Hague) to the coastal villages next to wide sandy beaches. I have visited many hospitals that provide excellent care, and I am impressed with the medical call centers that triage sick from less sick persons and make GP appointments.

History. Prior to World War II, a patchwork of small insurance initiatives through unions and workplaces provided basic coverage of physician visits. After the war, health care insurance was required with government regulation of prices.

Prices for medical care. Determined through negotiations between the insurers, hospitals, physicians, and others, with advice from the National Health Care Institute. Some prices are freely negotiated; others are set at a national standard rate.

Insurance. All persons are required to buy basic private insurance, which costs about $150 per month ($1,800 a year). This provides 40% of funding. Additional revenue comes from employer taxes (50%) and general taxes (10%). There are several large nonprofit insurance companies regulated by the government. Optional insurance is generally not needed because basic insurance covers all medical care, except eyeglasses, prescriptions, and co-pays.

Maximum out-of-pocket cost per person per year. Out-of-pocket costs are about $500 per person per year.

Access to care. Access to medical care is excellent. People can call their GP directly for an appointment or call a regional call center for advice and appropriate referral.

- GPs: Appointments from the same day to a week.
- Specialists: Patients are seen the same day up to weeks, depending on the urgency.
- Emergency care: Emergency departments are similar to US ED specialists. The standard European number 112 connects a

person to a regional call center, which employs medical technicians, nurses, and physicians. The regional call center can do everything from dispatch an ambulance to advise persons on home care. After hours GPs are located at most hospitals, adjacent to EDs, and care by the GP is free for those persons with basic insurance. However, if a person is triaged or demands care in the actual ED, a co-pay of $100 EU is charged.

Hospitals. Holland has 90 nonprofit hospitals. A government-organized committee sets charges for hospitals and physicians.

Finland

Finland is a small country of 5.5 million people located in the far north; most of the country is north of latitude 60 degrees, similar to the state of Alaska. In my contact with physicians and hospitals, I found the medical care to be excellent. I have had many detailed discussions with physicians and visited hospitals in Helsinki, Espoo, and Kuopio.

History. A municipal and regional system of health care was developed after independence from Russia in December 1917. An expanded role of the national government developed after World War II that set standards. Each of the 295 municipalities in cooperation with 19 regions is responsible for organizing a health care system for its residents. Think of this as if each US county and state was required to organize and provide health care to its residents.

Prices for medical care. Prices are set by the local government. A GP visit is in the range of $25–$35, $35–$50 for a specialist, and $60 for an ED visit. The hospital daily charge is in the $50 range, and drug prices vary. Hospitals in turn bill the local government, but the fees billed are a fraction of US charges. I estimate that a $5,000 charge to visit an ED in the United States might be billed to the local Finnish county government for around $500, with a $60 patient co-pay.

Insurance. As in Great Britain, there is no cost for universal health care in Finland; it is funded through taxes. People may also purchase private insurance. Some large companies may also provide insurance that permits employees to be seen at private physician offices, which account for about 4% of medical outpatient care.

Maximum out-of-pocket cost per person per year. For the public system, it is about $800 for medical care and hospital care, plus $600 for prescription medicines. Once the maximum out-of-pocket threshold is reached, a person has no additional costs.

Access to care. Since health care is decentralized by region, each municipality sets up its health centers and hospitals following the rules of the central government. People are required to call or visit their local health center for urgent problems. They can call 1-1-2 for true emergencies and other numbers for advice and direction to health centers.

- GPs: In a public system, a person can call a GP directly for an appointment or travel to a health center (the US equivalent of urgent care) and be referred to a GP, an ED, or a specialist as determined by the triage nurse. For less urgent or routine problems, a person may wait days or several weeks. In the private system, one can make an appointment online within a few days or have same-day treatment at a walk-in private urgent care center.
- Specialists: In the public system, referral times depend on the acuity of the problem. As in the United States, it may take only days or be as long as weeks to see a specialist. Private appointments can be obtained the same day or within a few days.
- Emergency care: In an emergency, call 1-1-2. The staff assesses the urgency of the problem and can dispatch an ambulance. Some EDs do not allow walk-in traffic from 8 a.m. to late afternoon. Persons with urgent problems must call 1-1-2 or go to a health center. ED care is similar to the United States with skilled physicians, state-of-the-art facilities, and advanced technology. The recognition of emergency medicine as a medical specialty has only occurred during the past few years, and

training programs have now been developed for physicians who want to exclusively work in EDs.

Hospitals. Finland has more than 60 hospitals, divided into university hospitals, central hospitals, and regional hospitals. It also has a dozen private hospitals. Public hospital admissions are through EDs and health centers, and daily hospital charges are about $60 a day, up to the annual maximum of $800.

Take-Home Lessons for the United States

America could reduce health care expenditures by half if it adopted one of the many European health care systems. It would be too much of a major leap for the United States to adapt the British National Health System model, nationalize all hospitals, and place physicians on a federal payroll. This would be akin to having a VA health system for the entire population. It could work but would be a long and difficult process to achieve. But other European systems offer solutions to the outrageous cost of health care in the United States.

Medicare for All

Many members of Congress have advocated for Medicare for All. The price-saving feature is that Medicare has a set fee schedule, which is one-half to one-third the cost of many retail prices charged by hospitals and physicians. Setting maximum fees and prices for medical and hospital care is the core reason European countries spend half of what the United States spends on health care. Medicare and most European countries both use a DRG method of determining the cost of care and setting the price that can be charged. Medicare would need to be modified so that Part B covers 100% of expenses, not just 80%. And prescription drug prices would need to be negotiated as in Europe. Medicare for All could be phased in by first lowering eligibility to persons aged 55 years and older and then over time phasing in other age ranges.

Adopt the Dutch System

Many European countries have health care systems with participation from private health plans, but with price controls and support for low-income persons. The Netherlands' health care system is the closest to the current structure in the United States. Employer contributions provide the largest portion of revenue. Private insurance companies are required to spend 95% of their premiums on health care. In Holland, no person is excluded from a health plan because of a preexisting condition. Maximum prices for hospital, physician, and other services are regulated in Holland. The United States could control prices by adapting the current Medicare fee schedules. Maximum charges for prescription drug prices would need to be set as in the Netherlands.

Bottom line: The US Congress must pass legislation that regulates charges and fees, in keeping with all systems of health care in Western Europe.

SIX

The Affordable Care Act of 2010 and Other Federal Health Care Laws

KEY CONCEPTS

1. Federal laws have shaped the delivery of health care in America.
2. The concept of government as a payer for civilian health care started with the Medicare Act of 1965.
3. Many federal laws intent on "doing good" for the people have loopholes that benefit corporations and increase health care costs.
4. In 2018, the health care industry spent more than a half a billion dollars on lobbying.
5. The Affordable Care Act 2010 provided protections for many Americans but ushered in increased profits for health plans and other sectors of the health care industry.

Corporations spent $380 million to influence the Affordable Care Act, also known as Obamacare.

Lobbyists for the health plan industry spent $86 million to influence Obamacare.

The health care sector made campaign contributions of $1.5 million to Senator Max Baucus (see discussion on Obamacare and Senator Baucus).

One of my first memories of the lobbying process at the US Congress was as a member of the Healthcare Committee at the annual "Cap-to-Cap" trip to Washington, DC, sponsored by the Sacramento Chamber of Commerce. As I rushed up and down the hallways of Senate and House office buildings to make a tight meeting schedule in my frumpy JCPenney wash-and-wear pants and old gray sports coat, I was shocked to see an army of professional lobbyists lining the hallways. And, unlike me, they were dressed in slick $2,000 suits, expensive polished black wing tip shoes, and gold Rolex watches.

"Who are these people?" I asked a colleague.

"They are the real lawmakers," he replied.

"What do you mean?" I said.

"They meet with members of Congress, and make their case for laws that increase the profit of their corporations. Then, the lobbyists take our elected officials to dinner, feed them more one-sided propaganda, and sweeten the deal; the corporations send congressional election campaigns big checks."

"So our own lobbying on overcrowded EDs may not have much impact," I replied.

"Yep."

Many actions and inactions of the US Congress have facilitated the evolution of our health care system from bedside medicine to corporate medicine. Federal laws have shaped and molded the health care delivery systems in America. A complete discussion of all the federal laws that affect our health care system is beyond the scope of this book. This chapter will address laws that have a major effect on the public health and the delivery of health care in America. Most important of these laws is the landmark Patient Protection and Affordable Care Act (ACA) of 2010, often referred to as Obamacare.

Some important laws that affect all Americans are as follows

1. *1906: The Pure Food and Drug Act.* This was one of the first laws to protect the public from illness and death from unsafe food and drugs. The act, Public Law 59-384, prohibited interstate and foreign traffic in adulterated or mislabeled food and drug products. This is considered to be one of the first consumer protection laws, which resulted from public outcry over conditions in the meat packing industry. *The Jungle* by Upton Sinclair exposed such conditions. This book was required reading when I attended high school and perhaps influenced my decision to pursue a career in medicine. The Food and Drug Administration evolved into a regulatory body in 1927 from the 1906 act.

2. *1938: The Food, Drug, and Cosmetic Act.* This law required additional safety for medications and strengthened the FDA's ability to enforce the law and required proof that new drugs were effective as claimed by the manufacturer. This law was discussed in chapter 1.

3. *1965: The Medicare Act.* Officially called the Health Insurance for the Aged and Disabled Act, it established both Medicare and Medicaid programs. These programs provided billions of federal dollars for health care services to certain groups of individuals, including people aged 65 and older and others meeting certain criteria. The details of how these programs work are described in chapter 4, "Health Plans."

From a health care policy standpoint, this was a landmark law. For the first time in history, the federal government would be paying private doctors and hospitals to care for millions of people. There was intense opposition by certain groups, including the American Medical Association. Ronald Regan worked as a spokesperson against Medicare, calling it socialized medicine, implying that it was a step toward communism.

The act was amended multiple times over the years, with some authority given to the federal agencies to make rules and regulations. Most important, the concept of diagnostic related group (DRG) was introduced. Under the DRG payment system, hospitals would be paid for a diagnosis such as pneumonia. The hospital would receive a set amount of dollars for caring for a patient with pneumonia. This would prevent a hospital from charging for every single bandage, pain pill, or special items to raise the bill and increase profits. The concept of DRGs has been widely adapted by European countries as noted in chapter 5.

4. *1973: The HMO Act.* This law encouraged the formation of health maintenance organizations. The intent of the legislation was to control health care costs while maintaining quality. However, unforeseen by the creators of the law, the creation of for-profit HMOs allowed corporations to make large profits by withholding needed medical care.

5. *1976: The Medical Device Amendments to the Food, Drug, and Cosmetic Act of 1938.* This law as well as others governing medical devices is discussed in chapter 8.

6. *1984: Hatch-Waxman Act.* As noted in chapter 1, the intent of the law was to encourage the pharmaceutical industry to increase

production of generic medications, presumably because they would cost less. It provided fast tracks for marketing of generics. But the legislation included many loopholes for a broad range of prescription drugs, allowed for extended patent protection, and increased corporate profits.

7. *1985: The Consolidated Omnibus Reconciliation Act (COBRA) Act.* This act contains many provisions, including some on health care. It expanded employer-based health care insurance by extending rights for temporary continuation of employer group health plan coverage for employees who leave their job for one of many reasons. Ex-employees must pay the entire cost for this coverage.

8. *1985: The Emergency Medicine Transfer and Labor Act.* This law was included in the 1985 COBRA previsions and changed the landscape of emergency departments by requiring that all persons with an emergency medical condition (EMC) would be provided care in EDs, regardless of insurance status or ability to pay. We will discuss this act in chapter 7, "Emergency Departments."

9. *1996: The Health Insurance Portability and Accountability Act of 1996 (HIPAA).* The intent of this act was to place safeguards on the flow of health care information. It places privacy requirements on personally identifiable health care records maintained by the health plans, hospitals, doctors, and other health care industries. Motivating factors include preventing computers to trade personal health information from one corporation to another, and to enhance doctor to doctor patient care related communication. To some extent, the latter intent has backfired, as an ED physician, I have been refused information from physicians even when caring for their patients in near death situations; "I can't tell you anything because of HIPAA." This 1996 act also expanded coverage of post employment COBRA health plan coverage.

10. *2003: The Medicare Prescription Drug Improvement and Modernization Act.* This law was sold to the public as a means of providing prescription drugs to Medicare recipients at an affordable price. It privatized the prescription drug functions of Medicare

Part D. Corporate lobbyists successfully included provisions that allowed Big Pharma to benefit by charging high prices to intermediary corporations. Distributors could charge high co-pays to patients and refuse to pay for some important drugs.

11. *2009: The HITECH Act.* The intent of this act was to bring the medical industry into the world of high-tech computerization and improve care through the use of the electronic medical record (EMR), also referred to as the electronic health record (EHR). However, this law resulted in physicians inputting data into complex computer systems, frustrating physicians, and reducing the number of patients that could be seen in a unit of time. It also required additional data added to the electronic medical record called *meaningful use.* As noted in chapter 3 on physicians, many physicians consider meaningful use data to be a waste of time, including myself.

12. *2010: The Affordable Care Act.* The remainder of this chapter will focus on the ACA (commonly referred to as Obamacare).

The Affordable Care Act of 2010

Many health care policy experts consider the ACA to be the most significant piece of federal health care legislation since the Medicare Act of 1965. Congress spent much of 2009 debating and revising the proposed ACA. Senator Max Baucus played a central role in negotiating the details of the ACA and making compromises between liberal Democrats and conservative Republicans. As noted at the beginning of the chapter, he also received generous campaign donations from corporations that wanted to ensure they received a piece of the pie. Key elements in Obamacare as originally proposed, such as the public option, had to be removed to get enough votes to get ACA passed. Even in early 2010, the outcome was placed in jeopardy when the Senate lost its 60 seat supermajority when Republican Scott Brown won the election for Ted Kennedy's seat in Massachusetts.

Only through skillful application of reconciliation rules were House and Senate leaders able to get the final ACA passed and signed into law by President Obama on March 23, 2010 (box 6.1).

Box 6.1

Key elements of the Affordable Care Act

1. Requires all persons to have health care insurance—the individual mandate.
2. Penalizes (with a monetary fine) persons who fail to have health insurance. Congress removed this element effective 2019.
3. Creates federal and state exchanges for persons to purchase insurance who do not have insurance provided by an employer, Medicare, Medicaid, Veterans Affairs, or the military.
4. Provides US government assistance to help pay for insurance for low-median income persons and families through the advance tax credit program.
5. Expands the federal Medicaid program to include very low or no-income persons or families.
6. Prohibits health plans from using preexisting conditions as a pretext to refuse or to increase prices.
7. Limits age-adjusted insurance rate spread to three times minimum to maximum.
8. Prohibits health plans from selling junk insurance.
9. Requires insurance plans to cover certain basic services.
10. Reaffirms use of the electronic medical record for physicians and hospitals.
11. Requires health plans to spend at least 80% of money collected on medical care (medical loss ratio).
12. Requires health plans to return excessive profits to consumers.
13. Provides direct government subsidies to insurance companies for providing health care insurance through government-run exchanges: the Bronze, Silver, Gold, Platinum plans.
14. Creation of accountable care organizations (ACOs). Requires groups of physicians and hospitals to unify and to create systems to reduce cost of care while improving quality.

A new Congress, with a Republican majority was sworn in in January 2011. Since then the House of Representatives voted over 50 times to repeal the ACA. A bill reached the floor of the US Senate in 2017, in which Obamacare narrowly escaped being overturned by a vote of 51–49. Nearly a decade after its passage, it continues to be discussed and hotly debated from Main Street diners and coffee shops to nationally televised presidential political debates.

The ACA was an extensive piece of legislation of nearly 2,300 pages. It required the Department of Health and Human Services to write rules and regulations, estimated at 16,000 to 20,000 pages.

Implementation of elements of the ACA were phased in over several years. A summary follows:

1. *Requires all persons to have health care insurance.* The mandate to require nearly everyone to have health care insurance was not in the original proposals of the ACA. However, the insurance industry lobbied Congress to include the mandate. The industry was concerned that healthy people would not sign up to buy insurance, leaving the industry on the hook to provide insurance to only high-risk groups. But requiring people to buy insurance (or to have insurance through other means) was felt by many in Congress to be unconstitutional and was a key reason for the multiple attempted repeals of the ACA. In December 2019, a federal appeals court struck down the requirement to buy health care insurance.

2. *Invokes monetary penalty for not having health care insurance.* A person who did not sign up with a health insurance plan faced a fine. Initially $75, this progressively increased to a 2.5% of income. The constitutionality of forcing people to buy health insurance was challenged in court and upheld by the Supreme Court in June 2012. However, in 2018, Congress repealed the penalty for not having health insurance, thus essentially eliminating the individual mandate. As of tax year 2019, there is no penalty for not having health insurance.

3. *Creates federal and state exchanges.* These exchanges allow persons to purchase health care insurance at a reasonable price. This group includes people who do not have insurance provided by an employer, Medicare, Medicaid, or the VA or military. Only about 10% of the US population falls into the group that needs to purchase on exchanges. The four standardized plans are Bronze, Silver, Gold, and Platinum. The plans that provide more comprehensive insurance are more expensive.

As noted in chapter 4 ("Health Plans"), many people complain about the least expensive Bronze level insurance. It carries a deductible of over $6,300 per person per year or $12,000 for the family plan. Until a person has forked $6,000 out of pocket, they may not get any health care paid for except for a few primary care doctor visits, often with co-pays ranging from $40 to $90. "It's like having no insurance," a patient told me. "Almost every charge is for me to pay." This lower tier was intended to be catastrophic, to save having a car or a home repossessed. Many people do not own a home, and their vehicle is "owned" by the bank that supplied the loan. But Bronze is all some families can afford.

4. *Provides federal assistance to purchase health care insurance.* The US government provides assistance (a subsidy) to pay for insurance purchased through government-controlled exchanges for individuals and families making less than $100,000. This is done on a sliding scale, which uses complicated formulas that consider

- Age of enrolled members
- Household size
- Income as a percent of federal poverty level (up to 400%)
- Income-based subsidy from the federal government

Example 1: John Smith, age 55, buys the Bronze health care plan to cover his family. The Bronze family plan costs $24,000 a year. The Smith family income is more than $140,000. John Smith pays the full $24,000; the federal government provides zero dollars in assistance.

Example 2A: Jill Boyd, age 31, plans to buy a Bronze health care plan. Her income is $31,000. The Bronze plan costs $6,000 for someone in her age group. The government subsidy for her income is $3,600 (provided as a tax credit). Jill's cost to buy the Bronze plan is $2,400.

Example 2B: Jill changes her mind and decides to buy the Silver plan. The Silver plan for her age costs $7,600 a year. Her government subsidy would be the same $3,600, but she would pay $4,000 a year for the Silver plan. The accounting to provide the federal subsidy is complex and involves year-end rectification through the individual's tax return to receive a tax credit. This is strange math: the tax credit has already been paid to the insurance company.

5. *Expands the federal Medicaid program.* The original Medicaid program provided health care insurance to a limited number of qualifying low-income groups. The ACA allows states to expand the pool of eligible people. In some states, large numbers of previously uninsured persons can now qualify for health care through Medicaid. In California, 33% of the population receives medical care through the Medicaid program.

6. *Eliminates preexisting conditions exclusion used by health plans.* This requirement prohibits health plans from using conditions as a pretext to refuse or increase insurance prices. Before the ACA, many insurance companies would charge substantially higher prices to persons with higher-risk medical problems, such as diabetes or hypertension. In some cases, patients were refused insurance outright. The ACA also eliminated the "dirty trick" of companies retroactively canceling insurance after a high claim for a hospitalization by finding out that a person did not disclose having certain medical conditions. Preexisting conditions, in some cases, included acne, common colds, or poison oak.

7. *Limits age-adjusted insurance rate spread to three times minimum to maximum.* Before the ACA, insurance companies would charge older persons higher premiums than younger persons. In some cases, older persons would pay 10 times the rates for younger persons. The ACA states that the maximum age rate can be no greater than three times that for younger persons.

8. *Prohibits insurance companies selling junk insurance.* Junk plans were inexpensive and therefore attractive to many people. Junk insurance is just that, junk. These plans provide minimal coverage and usually come with loopholes. A plan may just cover primary care doctor visits but not hospitalization. Or a plan may pay $25,000 in medical expenses, which is not much when a hospitalization requiring intensive care could cost $200,000. Or the plan may have a larger set amount, say, $50,000 in coverage but exclude

visits to EDs and specialists or not pay for CT scans or MRIs. In late 2018, the Trump administration proposed allowing certain forms of junk insurance to be sold again.

9. *Requires insurance plans to cover certain essential services.* This element in the law was in response to the junk insurance business. Examples of essential items that must be included in health plans include maternity and newborn care, mental health services, emergency services, prescription drugs, and hospitalization.

10. *Expands use of the electronic medical record (EMR) by physicians and hospitals.* As noted earlier in this chapter, the EHR requirement was made law with the HITECH act of 2009. The EHR placed additional requirements for data collection on physicians and hospitals.

11. *Requires health plans to spend at least 80% of money collected on medical care.* The intent of this section of the ACA is to reduce huge profits and encourage efficiency. Health plans must spend 80% of what they collect in premiums on actual medical care. The amount spent on actual medical care has the confusing term *medical loss* attached to it. Plans such as Medicare have a medical loss ratio of 95%; health plans in European countries also have a medical loss of close to 95%.

12. *Requires health plans to return excessive profits to consumers.* Certain health plans are allowed to retain only 20% of total premiums (money collected for profit and administration). If health plans keep more for themselves, they must return it to the plan members. Health plan XYZ collects $100 billion and spends $70 billion on medical care. It must return $10 billion to the policyholders at the end of the year. Keep in mind that most European insurance companies and the US agency that administers Medicare retain 5% or less.

13. *Provides direct government subsidies to certain health plans.* To help insurance companies support passage of the ACA, the cost-sharing reduction program was added for start up years 2014–2016. The purpose was to directly subsidize the Silver, Gold, and Platinum plans, thus making their sticker price more affordable to

persons buying health insurance on the government-run exchanges. Congress beginning in 2014, refused to fund the program, and President Trump used an executive order to terminate this program. However, in April 2020, the US Supreme Court reinstated the program.

14. *Creation of accountable care organizations.* Many, including the author, poorly understand this well-intended element in the ACA. The goal is to encourage groups of physicians and hospitals to determine how to reduce the cost of care by reducing redundancy in unneeded testing, procedures, and exams. Successful affordable care organizations are rewarded with extra federal dollars (a small fraction of the total savings) to doctors and hospitals.

The Influence of the Health Care Industry on US Health Care Policy, Law, and Economics

The health care industry spends millions of dollars each year to influence Congress. During the writing of the ACA, lobbying by the health care industry was intense and resulted in shaping the ACA to ensure continuing profits for the health care industry. Health plans now receive billions of additional dollars because of the federal mandate that requires everyone to have insurance. In addition, generous federal subsidies further increase profits. Other for-profit health plans that administer Medicaid programs have received increased profits because of the Medicaid expansion. In California, nearly a third of the population—12 million people—has Medicaid coverage.

Why were not drug prices aggressively addressed by the ACA? As we discussed in chapter 1, industry groups such as Big Pharma have enormous influence over Congress, much more than average citizens. The ACA could have provided a framework to reduce drug prices through negotiations, but Big Pharma successfully defeated proposals to reduce prescription drug costs. The public, along with physicians, hospitals, and insurance companies all want lower prescription drug prices.

Health Care Corporation Spend Huge Sums of Money to Lobby Congress

The entire health care industry spent over $500 million just in 2018, with estimates of $556 million. There are 2,800 lobbyists for 435 voting members of Congress. Money spent by sector of health care obtained from the OpenSecrets.org follows:

- Pharmaceuticals and health products: $280,134,421
- Hospitals and nursing homes: $99,649,413
- Health professionals: $89,555,000
- Health plans: $79,538,000
- Other: $7,000,000

This intense degree of lobbying means that our representatives and senators listen to an endless stream of one-sided persuasion to enact laws or create loopholes to benefit the profits of the health care industry. I have seen some of these slick handouts and glossy brochures passed out by lobbyists. They are written to present only one side of an argument—the side that benefits the profits for the health care industry. And they are cleverly written to convey the message that industry is devoted to the good health of the average person on Main Street.

Bribes to Congress—Some Hidden, Some Not

During the 2018 election cycle, the health care industry gave $225 million in campaign donations to federal candidates, including incumbents and challengers. While by law, there can be no strings attached, there is an implied, "You make us happy, and we'll be there for you at the next election." When I was a candidate for Congress in 2016, I learned that campaigns are expensive to run. To be successful, or even to have a chance in competitive races, the candidate needs money, lots of it, as much as $3 million or $4 million for each campaign. And US House members face elections every two years. Getting large sums of campaign dollars seems easier compared to collecting individual $25 donations.

For this reason, many congressional candidates have not refused industry funding. In exchange, industry will want to set up a friendly meeting with a lobbyist and the elected congressperson. Campaign donations come with an implied "I get access to Congress." Access means lobbying for laws and loopholes that result in profit. In the case of health care, profit is most likely at the expense of us paying through high co-pays, deductibles, surprise medical bills, higher taxes, higher drug prices, and higher costs of goods and services. After all, employers pay the lion's share of employer-based health care insurance.

We are fortunate to have OpenSecrets reports on lobbying and direct campaign contributions. That's where the hard data I reported previously came from. But there is also dark money, unlimited sums of dollars from persons or companies whose identity can be hidden through dummy companies. Super PACs are not the traditional political action committees that have $5,000 donation limits.

Super PACs either support or don't support a candidate. They were legitimized by the US Supreme Court's *Citizens United* ruling in 2010, which treated political donations as protected speech. Super PACs have no restrictions on how much money they can collect or spend and vague reporting on sources of income. Super PACs are required not to coordinate or cooperate with the candidate's campaign (committee).

But members of Congress know about these super PACs, and many know how to vote to continue to receive super PAC support in the next election.

Bottom line: The best solution to improve health care at less cost is to limit corporate influence on members of Congress by restricting lobbying and by enacting effective campaign finance reform.

SEVEN

Emergency Departments

KEY CONCEPTS

1. Federal law requires that all people presenting to emergency departments be evaluated.
2. Overcrowding in EDs results in long waits for minor problems.
3. Corporations exercise increasing control of ED physicians.
4. Hospital charges for care may be very high and not covered by insurance.

Campaign contributions to congressional candidates and lobbying of Congress by hospitals that have EDs during 1990–2020: hundreds of millions of dollars.

Campaign contributions to congressional candidates by the American College of Emergency Physicians during 1990–2020: $14 million

What stands out in my mind from a 30-year career as an emergency department (ED) doctor? Overcrowding. And long waiting times and overcrowding continue to get worse. In almost every state and city, there are too many sick and injured people crowded into too few beds, exceeding capacity. Support services, including laboratory, simple x-ray, and advanced imaging, are congested and delayed. Hospital beds are frequently totally filled, resulting in admitted patients spending hours (sometimes days) in crowded and noisy ED hallways before being taken upstairs to a real hospital bed. I have written extensively on overcrowding, with over 20 peer-reviewed publications, but little has changed to make EDs less crowded. I also remember being totally exhausted at the end of my 12-hour shifts but happy for the people I helped.

I have also seen so many improvements in the quality of medical and trauma care in EDs. Skilled physicians using advanced procedures and drugs save patients who are within minutes of death. Antidotes are available for nearly every type of poisoning; a wide array of testing helps in the diagnosis of even the most confusing symptoms.

Over the past 40 years, EDs have evolved from triage and first aid stations to sophisticated, state-of-the-art acute diagnostic and treatment units. The small treatment room of the past on the first floor of the hospital has grown into an essential component of the American health care system that provides care for over 120 million visits annually. Some hospitals that had small two-room EDs have transformed into 60-room EDs.

Recall in chapter 3, I described an injury to one of my fingers when I was 10 years old that was quickly treated in a local public clinic. If this injury had occurred in the present day, my mom would have driven me to the hospital ED. The waiting room would have been filled with people. We would have waited in line to see the triage nurse, who would have told my mom that a splinter was low priority. The nurse would have wondered why we hadn't called our doctor or visited an urgent care center. If my mother had called the doctor's office, she would have been told that the next available appointment would be the next day, and she would have had to call urgent care. A busy urgent care would have referred her to the ED.

In this hypothetical scenario, we would have waited many hours in the ED waiting room (from 2 to 12 hours) before being called back by a nurse and taken to an exam bed. The exam space would be a narrow gurney with clean sheets, but perhaps with dried blood splattered on the rails and separated from 12 other gurneys by flimsy curtains. I would hear other patients moaning and groaning in pain within feet of me. A nurse would then ask my mother a hundred questions about my immunizations, child abuse, seat belts, diet, drugs, smoking (yes, even as a kid), alcohol, depression, and on and on.

Help. I just want the big splinter out and not to feel like I was on a quiz show! After another hour, a rushed and frazzled physician would examine me, and say, "We'll pull the splinter out and you'll be good as new." But, first, they'd need to order a "splinter tray" with the instruments needed for the splinter removal, another hour. Finally, with the splinter removed, we'd go home some six or eight hours after arrival to the ED. A few weeks later a $380 bill would arrive in the mail for physician services. Two months later a second bill of $4,600 for hospital ED charges would arrive. Can anyone argue that current care is better and more cost efficient than 50 years ago?

The Evolution of Emergency Departments

The dramatic changes that have occurred in EDs are akin to the transition from the horse and buggy to the automobile. The reasons are complex and multifactorial. First, emergency medicine has become recognized as its own specialty, concurrent with advances in technology, and increasing demands for care in the ED. American culture has evolved together with public expectations for 24/7 medical care. The television series *ER* staring George Clooney helped increase awareness of the important role EDs serve in our health care system. Hospitals saw enormous growth of people receiving care at EDs and a chance to increase revenue and profit.

Types of Emergency Departments
Teaching Hospital Emergency Departments

Teaching hospital EDs are located in large cities, and most are affiliated with medical schools. Yes, there were some exceptions. EDs were staffed with young enthusiastic, newly minted physicians: interns and residents. Collectively called house staff, the ED was the melting pot for rotation interns, residents in internal medicine, surgery, anesthesia, and practically every other specialty. The sickest patients in a city usually came by ambulance to teaching hospitals. Patients who had no money came too, and many were very sick.

Add the medical students, of which I was one, to the wild and chaotic environment in 1974. I got my fill of experience at the San Francisco General Hospital ED and had plenty of patients to practice sewing up lacerations, placing splints and casts, starting IVs, giving IV and intermuscular medications, and ordering any x-rays and laboratory work. After I figured out what was wrong with a patient, I'd discuss it with an intern or a resident. Senior doctors only appeared if a famous person came into the ED as a patient. The free-for-all atmosphere was great for teaching students and interns responsibility and the art of applying the science of medicine. Did we make mistakes? Sure we did. But, at the time, we thought we were too smart to make errors. Until something major went wrong, the hospital administration and major departments paid little attention to what went on in ED.

What changed in teaching hospitals? Between 1980 and 2000, the staffing in teaching EDs changed and the quality of care improved. Fewer residents rotated through the ED from specialties such as anesthesia, surgery, medicine, pediatrics, family practice, and obstetrics and gynecology. In their place came residents in emergency medicine, whose focus and training was just that: emergency medicine. Teaching hospitals hired full-time expert specialists in emergency medicine called attending physicians. Every patient now gets evaluated early on by an attending. Teaching hospitals gave birth to a new recognized specialty—emergency medicine—beginning in the 1980s. The details of the establishment of the specialty of emergency medicine are described later in this chapter. Many university teaching hospital EDs have developed advanced care for critical time-dependent conditions and have received special certifications, including as trauma centers, stroke centers, and heart centers.

Community Hospital Emergency Departments

Forty years ago, community hospitals historically were less crowded and much quieter than teaching hospitals. In many hospitals, the EDs were just that, a room on the ground floor of the hospital. Long ago, there was no ED doctor on duty. When a patient appeared, the ED nurse would call the patient's physician (usually a general practitioner). If the patient had not seen a physician recently, the nurse would call an on-call physician. The physician would instruct the nurse to (1) send the patient over to their office, (2) admit the patient to the hospital (a physician would give admission orders over the phone), or (3) expect the physician to arrive immediately, at lunch, or after office hours.

As time progressed, EDs became busier. At the same time, more patients had no identified general practitioner, primary care doctor, or other private physician. On-call physicians to the ED became overwhelmed. So larger hospitals hired physicians to staff the EDs 24 hours a day to handle the patient volume. Initially, hospitals were not choosy about who they hired; anyone with a medical license would be hired to "cover" the ED. Who were these pioneer ED physicians? They were a mix of physicians in training (residents) who had just received their medical license, physicians who dropped out of residencies, and physicians from almost any specialty who wanted to make a few extra bucks. Few worked full time in EDs and hence a term evolved for part-timers working in EDs—*moonlighters*.

I was one of these moonlighters. In those early days, working 24-hour-long shifts meant grabbing a catnap in the middle of the night, but only when things slowed down. At times, I was overwhelmed. At one small hospital in the small California foothill town of Placerville, they had a solution to ED overcrowding. Borrowing from the recent days of bedside medicine, I could call in a local general or family practice physician to work a six-hour shift, side by side with me. These local practicing physicians helped to teach me the art of medicine: fewer laboratory tests and x-rays and next-day follow-up in a local primary care physician's office, regardless of insurance.

As time progressed, more and more people needed ED care. The pool of physicians willing to work in EDs was not large enough to meet the demand. Hospital administrators saw that physicians with special training in emergency medicine provided better care for patients with acute, undiagnosed illness. Hospitals also recognized the advantage to having full-time physicians dedicated to emergency departments from medical, legal, and malpractice standpoints. Larger hospitals needed double coverage—that is, two or more ED physicians working side by side at the same time. To help fill the demand, new university-trained emergency medicine specialists were hired. ED physicians treat and stabilize injuries and illnesses but cannot admit patients to the hospital. When a patient needed admission from the ED, the ED physician would call the patient's primary care physician or, in the case of a patient who had no PCP, an on-call or an admitting physician, from a list usually posted on the wall of their workstation. Now, a hospitalist performs these functions (see chapter 3).

The Federal Law Changed Emergency Departments Forever

The Emergency Medicine Transfer and Labor Act (EMTALA) had a major effect on the way EDs did business. In the past, persons with very serious emergencies could be denied care in EDs and turned away. In the early 1980s, a man once presented to a hospital ED with signs of a heart attack and was told to take a bus to a county hospital. This is no longer allowed.

EMTALA was signed into law as part of the Consolidated Omnibus Reconciliation Act of 1985 and is referred to as COBRA in some older ED literature. The intent of this act was to prevent persons with true emergencies from being denied care and turned away from the ED. The legislation grew out of a practice in the early 1980s by some hospital EDs of requiring potential patients to show evidence of insurance before receiving care. This requirement resulted in unnecessary pain, suffering, and even death. In some cases, ambulances with sick or injured patients were turned away from private hospitals and directed to a county hospital. Other patients were seen briefly in EDs and then sent across town to a county or university hospital ED just because they had no money. These transfers were referred to in the press and medical literature as *dumps*, hence EMTALA is referred to by some as *anti-dumping* legislation.

I remember caring for patients in the ED as an intern who arrived by ambulance from community hospitals with baggage tags attached to their toes. On these tags were cryptic notes with words like "needs detox," "admit for pneumonia," and "rule out heart attack."

The key element in EMTALA is that all persons presenting to EDs must have a medical screening exam to determine whether they have an emergency medical condition. If they do have a condition that could be an emergency, such as chest pain, abdominal pain, high fever, and bleeding, then they must be stabilized in the ED. To stabilize means to provide medical and surgical treatment to prevent bodily harm. EMTALA was later amended to include psychiatric conditions and women in labor.

The financial impact of EMTALA resulted in EDs providing care but not being paid. This has been offset in part by special funds from the federal government, so-called Disproportionate Share Hospital (DSH) payments. In addition, some believe that EMTALA has resulted in ED crowding as persons without money or insurance can get free medical care.

Overcrowding in Emergency Departments

In the past, with the exception of urban teaching hospitals, EDs were not crowded and waits for care were short. Then EDs began to become overcrowded and waits to be seen grew very long, with some waits of more than 12 hours. I served as an expert in a legal case in which a patient was sent to a community hospital ED with a diagnosis of appendicitis and sat in the waiting room vomiting and in pain for 12 hours before being seen by a physician. His appendix ruptured during that 12-hour wait. Crowding in EDs first came to national attention in the early 1990s with a few professional journals describing the problem. Since then several hundred articles have been written on ED crowding and published in peer-reviewed publications.

As noted above, patients may have poor outcomes because of long wait times in EDs. Articles in our professional journals not only describe poor outcomes, but also the causes and effects of overcrowding and offer solutions. The solutions have not been easy, and many proposed changes to reduce crowding are expensive and difficult to implement. Reasons for overcrowding identified by articles in the emergency medicine literature include the following:

1. EDs and hospitals are too small to meet the demands of large numbers of patients.
2. Many patients have nowhere else to go for medical care, especially after hours. As noted in chapter 3, independent small

office primary care physicians are vanishing and corporate hospital based clinics have not made up the shortfall.

3. Patients receive detailed diagnostic workups (e.g., laboratory testing, x-rays, CT scans, MRIs).
4. Initial stabilization and treatment of sick patients are now done in the ED instead of in a hospital inpatient unit.
5. The population as a whole has more complex diseases.

My colleagues and I proposed several solutions for the problem of ED crowding in an article published in 2008: "Ten Solutions for Emergency Department Crowding." These included the following:

1. Expanding hospital capacity
2. Ending rules that result in hospital inefficiency
3. Providing care to patients with only true emergencies
4. Providing alternatives for primary care for the uninsured and underinsured
5. Stopping boarding admitted patients in the ED
6. Using evidence-based guidelines to limit overutilization of imaging
7. Changing admitting patterns
8. Expanding the role of ancillary personnel
9. Calling the nurse first (see chapter 5, "European Systems of Health Care Delivery")
10. Preventing injuries and disease

Establishment of the Specialty of Emergency Medicine

In the past, any licensed physician, no matter what their specialty, could work in EDs. In teaching hospitals, EDs were divided into separate areas based on specialty—for example, an ED could be split into a surgical unit, a medical unit, an obstetrics and gynecology unit, and a pediatric unit, each organized and operated by physicians of the respective specialty. Now most EDs are one unit, with emergency medicine specialists who have been trained in the acute aspects of each of the specialty areas.

It became evident in the 1980s that the ability to quickly diagnose a wide range of disease and injury symptoms required special knowledge. A surgeon would not be able to rapidly diagnose and treat new onset diabetic ketoacidosis as well as a physician who did it every day. Likewise, an endocrinologist might have difficulty diagnosing a spleen ruptured in a car crash. The physicians who did work full time in EDs began to describe new methods of acute evaluation in peer-reviewed journals. The ED approach was that minutes matter. Areas where no established specialty was considered expert, such as poisoning, snakebite, heatstroke, and drowning, soon became the domain of ED physicians. The most common presenting complaints of patients to the ED included chest pain, abdominal pain, and vomiting. Treating these problems required quick thinking that crossed the barriers of many specialties.

Efforts to train new physicians to work exclusively in EDs began in earnest in the 1980s. Three- or four-year residency training programs were created that provided the knowledge to save lives where minutes mattered. I started a training program at UC Davis in 1990, and it had taken three years to lay the groundwork, find funding, and obtain approval from the hospital, the medical school, and national credentialing agencies. Nationally, from 1980 to 2000, over 120 new residency training programs in emergency medicine were created.

Advanced technology is often used hand-in-hand with the emergency medicine specialty. In the past, only simple laboratory tests and x-rays were ordered in the ED. For example, three types of x-rays: chest x-rays, abdominal x-rays, and skull films accounted for most of the x-rays ordered in the ED. Now dozens of lab tests and sophisticated imaging from complex x-rays to MRIs, CT scans, and angiography are routinely ordered in the ED and done immediately. Some have termed this *one-stop shopping*. All these studies take time and have contributed to longer evaluation times in the ED and hence more crowding. The magic of advanced technology outweighs the disadvantage. Complex and difficult symptoms can now be quickly diagnosed. Once the proper diagnosis is made, the proper treatment can be started.

Similar to other areas of health care, these major advances in diagnosis and treatment have occurred in the ED since the 1980s. Lives have been saved and patients have been spared from painful, disabling conditions by quick and immediate treatments. But the charges for these services have far outstripped the actual costs. As a rule of thumb, the actual cost of advanced health care delivery is far less than what hospitals bill. Remember that Medicare payments are about one-third the charges billed by hospitals, and Medicare payments actually allow for hospitals to make a fair profit. And recall that European hospital EDs provide the same level of advanced care as in the United States.

The Emergency Department as the Portal of Hospital Admissions

Thirty years ago, a primary care physician or specialist physician would admit the patient directly to a bed in the hospital from their office. Now sick patients are sent to the ED, where they have a battery of tests and are then admitted. Community physicians, who in the past would see their own patients in the ED, now delegate that duty to the ED physician.

The Emergency Department as a Money Machine for Wall Street

Investors and large corporations largely ignored the ED until recently. Now it is viewed as an area of the hospital where millions of dollars of profit can be made from hospital and physician charges. As a result of the transition to staffing EDs 24/7 with physically present doctors, the dedicated ED doctor was born and issues related to newly forming physician ED groups arose.

Hospital Charges for ED Care

Thirty years ago, charges for ED care were affordable. Hospital administrators did not think of EDs as portals to a hospital admission for sick persons, or elective admissions, but only as first-aid stations. Up until about 1990, charges to patients and insurers for ED treatment were relatively inexpensive.

When I was appointed chief of emergency medicine at UC Davis in 1985, the total charge to a patient to be treated in our ED was limited to a $100 registration fee. No matter how sick or injured you were, or how long you stayed in the ED, no matter how many drugs and IVs, x-rays, or lab tests you received, your cost was only $100. As an aside, we had an observation area in the ED where we could keep people up to five days. And even if you could not pay, no one ended up homeless under a bridge as a result of a $100 medical bill. Low ED fees were true in many hospitals, where charges for evaluation and treatment in the ED were nominal. Hospitals would charge a nominal facility use fee, in the hundreds of dollars. This fee included all supplies, IVs, and medications.

One of my first assignments in 1986 at the university was to develop a billing system, both for the physician part of the bill and one for the hospital. In California, doctors must bill separately from hospitals. We worked with the lab and x-ray department to add in some of their charges. Even then, the maximum a person would be charged for care in the ED was about $1,000. But the hospital thought that was great; they just increased their billings by 10-fold with several strokes of the pen. Currently, ED charges for an evaluation for abdominal pain can be as high as $20,000. The facility use fee alone (i.e., the charge for lying on a gurney) could be as much as $6,000 (Hsia 2014).

Hospital fees and charges are separate from the physician's professional fee. In addition to the facility use fee, nearly every bandage, gauze pad, and towel carries a charge. And the facility use fees have jumped into the thousands of dollars. In addition, some hospitals charge a trauma activation fee for patients who have sustained injuries in auto crashes and other forms of trauma.

I have reviewed many hospital ED bills. Here is an example of one for a person involved in a minor auto crash, who arrived at the hospital by ambulance:

ED facility use fee	$6,800
Trauma activation charge	$5,000
Lab studies	$1,200
Imaging (radiology department)	$6,500
Supplies	$2,300
IV starts/blood draws	$200
Total	$22,200

The charge far exceeds the actual cost. How much profit is in the $22,200? It varies by institution, but profit could be in excess of $15,000. Sounds like a good investment for Wall Street investors. These numbers do not include physician fees from the ED physician and radiologist.

Physician Charges Professional Fees

Historically, a physician who provided care in the ED would send the patient a bill for the professional fee. Increasingly, the physician does not send a bill as an independent entity, but a corporation sends the bill in the name of the physician. It is important to understand how small groups of doctors who functioned independently became employees of large corporations and the cogs in the wheels of Wall Street business designed to make money from people seeking ED care. In the 1980s, community hospital administrators did not want the chore of scheduling and coordinating a ragtag army of ED moonlighters. Not infrequently, an ED doctor would not show up, and a private community physician would have to cover the ED. To complicate matters further, some states did not allow hospitals to employ physicians, requiring that physicians bill separately for services (and still do). The solution: find a willing moonlighter to take on the full-time responsibility of hiring, and scheduling ED docs. Some hospitals would help the new ED groups set up billing and even provide a subsidy to the ED group. There were usually one or two physicians who formed the ED physician groups, and they became the group's director doctors.

I was on the front line of the evolution of ED physician groups. I was invited to be the medical director and vice president of a new group a friend of mine set up in the 1980s to provide ED coverage in a hospital. In the end, I chose to stay in academics and missed the chance to amass millions of dollars as an ED group director. But I never regret my decision to remain a professor and to have the opportunity of organizing a residency training program in emergency medicine and help create the specialty of emergency medicine.

"The Corporate Practice of Emergency Medicine" (2019) is an article posted on the website of the American Academy of Emergency Physicians (AAEM). Robert McNamara, MD, professor and chair of emergency medicine at Temple University and former president of the AAEM, authored the article. He has written and lectured extensively on the topic of problems for patients and physicians related to mergers of small or single hospital physician groups into national mega Wall Street corporations. Problems include high fees and profits going to the corporation, the potential to have employment terminated for complaining about unsafe conditions, and pressure by the corporation to order unnecessary testing and hospital admission.

Some of these issues were the topic of Jim Keaney's book *The Rape of Emergency Medicine* (1992). The business model works like this (hypothetical dollar amounts): The director doctor of the group hires and pays doctors (called *scrubs*) $100 an hour to work 12- or 24-hour shifts in the ED. The director doctor controls the group's billing unit and collects fees from patients the scrubs cared for at a much higher rate, say, $200 an hour. The director doctor keeps the remaining $100 an hour, totaling up to $2,400 a day, for sitting in the kitchen scheduling shifts and hiring doctors to fill in shifts. That's the simple version of the book.

In many cases, the director doctor invites other doctors to become partners and form a management team (referred to as *suits*). The suits determine methods to maximize billings and collections for the group. Soon the scrubs are generating $300 an hour for the group but are still getting paid $100 an hour. Successful ED group suits then go to neighboring hospitals and get additional contracts, promising "better care by better doctors" than what these other hospitals had at that time. Growth of ED physician groups result in more money, more power, and clout to grow even bigger—just like other segments of American business.

At some point, Wall Street investors became interested. They bought up many ED groups (paying suits big dollars) and, ultimately, controlled contracts to provide ED care at dozens (in some cases, hundreds) of hospitals, employing hundreds of ED doctors. So, a portion of the professional fee paid by patients finds its way to Wall Street corporations. Besides sending ED patients maximum-sized bills, groups could control the behavior of scrubs that threatened the hospital–ED group contract. Scrubs who complained to the hospital about unsafe conditions could be silenced with a threat of being fired by the group (McNamara 2013).

Major corporate entities (including privately owned companies) that staff EDs with physicians include Envision, EmCare, and Team Health. These firms collectively provide ED physician services at hundreds of hospital EDs. A May 2018 article in *Forbes* describes an exorbitant fee of $2,255 for service by an Envision ED physician at a Florida ED it staffs (Kincaid 2018). The *New York Times* published a story on EmCare fees in an ED in Spokane, Washington. The company increased the highest level of physician care fee from $467 to $1,649. In addition, the number of patients billed at that highest level increased from 6% to 28% (Creswell 2017).

There are exceptions to this corporate evolution of ED physician groups. Some groups have remained small staffing only one community hospital, some groups include all the physicians as partners (referred as democratically run groups), and some groups refuse to be bought out by Wall Street or national chains.

Increasing Profits for Health Plans by Not Paying for ED Care

In the past, health plans would pay for ED care, minus a small deductible. In the 1990s, health plans determined that too many people were going to EDs for nonemergency conditions. The actual scientific studies showed only 10%–15% of patients had nonemergent conditions, and these persons had no means of knowing that their symptoms were not an emergency. How does the average person distinguish between the acute severe chest pain of indigestion and a heart attack?

The so-called retroactive denial of payment became a big issue, and emergency medicine professional organizations took their cause to Congress as well as to state legislative bodies. The bad press that the insurance corporations received from the public outcry was enough for them to temporarily back off and pay for most ED visits. But then again in 2016, health plans began refusing to pay for certain ED visits, an issue that was brought to the attention of Congress.

Solutions

Many issues regarding emergency departments were discussed in this chapter. Listed below are what I consider solutions to the most serious problems.

Crowding. Some of the solutions to ED crowding were discussed in this chapter. Foremost among solutions is to make 24/7 care available elsewhere for everyone, meaning equal access to primary and urgent medical care that would result with health care reform legislation. This includes financial support to independent primary care physicians, expanding their office hours, expanding urgent care clinics, and lifting restrictions for access placed by health plans.

Charges and prices. Outrageous prices should be addressed by setting maximal prices that EDs can charge, which has been done successfully in Europe. Medicare already sets maximum fees for patients. Some states have passed legislation that prohibits EDs from charging uninsured patients more than 125% of the Medicare rate. Why not apply that to everyone? Is it ethically right for a hospital to charge a patient with abdominal pain $6,000 "bed rent" just to lay on a gurney in a noisy hallway?

Protect emergency physicians. Emergency physicians should be able to practice without fear of termination for not following corporate protocols designed to make profit, must be allowed due process, and not feel threatened by noncompete contracts.

Require health plans to pay for care delivered in EDs. Prohibit retroactively denying payment by claiming the patient's medical or traumatic problem was not an emergency medical condition.

Bottom line: As discussed in other chapters, the US Congress must pass legislation to fix the many problems related to EDs and not have reform measures blocked by corporate entities.

EIGHT

The Medical Implant Device Industry

KEY CONCEPTS

1. Medical device implants are a $300 billion a year industry.
2. Devices have improved the quality of life for many recipients.
3. Many devices have a high profit margin.
4. Safety testing of some devices is lax.
5. Loopholes in device safety laws enacted by Congress have resulted in use of unsafe and harmful devices.

ABC News reported that, in 2017 and 2018, the medical device industry spent $36 million on lobbying.

OpenSecrets reported the 2018 cycle contributions to Congressional Campaigns by the Medical supply industry exceeded $5 million.

I remember watching *The Six Million Dollar Man*, a weekly TV drama depicting an injured US astronaut with secret bionic implants inserted into his body. These implants gave him superhuman strength, with muscle, brain, nerve, and eye capabilities that he used to fight evil. This popular 1970s TV series lasted five seasons. I was in medical school at that time—fresh out of my anatomy course. I concluded that *The Six Million Dollar Man* was pure fiction, and those implants were just a Dick Tracy dream. Nearly fifty years later, we have had an explosion of bionic implants. Implants are now a $300 billion industry, far beyond what could be imagined in the 1970s, and even more surprising, they are becoming available to most Americans. Implants improve the quality of life for many people but have not enabled the superhuman capabilities described in the TV show.

Implants are usually cataloged as medical devices. Loosely defined, medical devices include all physical objects used in medical and surgical care. In my everyday practice, I use a stethoscope, wooden tongue depressors, syringes, cutting blades, needle holders, and suture material. Emergency departments use ultrasound, intubation equipment, and devices to stabilize fractures. These are considered medical devices and are not discussed in this chapter. This chapter also will not talk about diagnostic visit–related equipment such as ultrasound or electrocardiogram (EKG) machines, or temporary external devices, such as splints and braces.

Many of my patients have medical implants. The most common implants people think of are hip, knee, and shoulder implants. These implants have given my patients renewed activity and mobility. The majority of people who have received joint implants do very well. However, a few patients develop complications. I have cared for patients with implant-related infections or deep venous thrombosis, requiring multiple return office visits. In the ED, I have also cared for patients who have had pacemakers fail or who have had their implanted joints dislocate. Almost daily I have cared for patients with coronary artery stents (tubes placed in coronary arteries to improve blood flow) and working heart pacemakers. Artificial eye lenses are very common in older people who have had surgery for cataracts, and I have placed and removed many intrauterine devices.

The device industry has lobbied Congress heavily and showered some in Congress with generous campaign donations. This influence has resulted in Congress failing to pass needed regulation, passing legislation with weak regulations, or passing legislation filled with loopholes that benefit industry. As a result, much safety testing is inadequate, and monopolies on products have driven up retail prices and increased profitability for Wall Street investors. History has shown that marketing of unsafe devices has harmed patients.

Implantable Devices: History and Evolution

Few implanted devices were commonly used before the 1940s. At that time, more orthopedic surgeons began using metal screws and plates to stabilize fractures. Decades before the Wall Street business model, perhaps this was the only "bedside medicine" application of implants. In the late 1950s and early 1960s, widespread applications of implantable devices were discovered. Cardiac pacemakers came to market, although the early models were wires implanted in the heart, with the actual battery-powered pacer placed outside the body. In addition to widespread use of orthopedic screws and plates, joint replacement became more widespread with hip joint replacement leading the way. Artificial heart valves were developed and saved many lives in those patients who had heart valve failure.

With our current corporate medicine, a mind-boggling number of patents are filed for implantable medical devices each year: thousands and thousands of patents for either totally new or look-alike devices are filed with the US Patent and Trademark Office. There is not just one type of artificial hip; there are many different types. The same for ear implants, insulin pumps, and artificial eye lenses.

As more devices came to market, Congress passed a number of laws supposedly to ensure safety. The laws addressed such safety questions as, Will an orthopedic screw rust and break? Will an artificial heart valve suddenly freeze up and stop blood flow? Do devices contain toxic substances, such as lead, cadmium, or mercury, that could leach into the body and cause harm? Notable federal legislation is discussed next.

1976: The Medical Device Amendments to the Food, Drug, and Cosmetic Act of 1938. The intent of this law is to provide reasonable assurance of the safety and effectiveness of medical devices. It does the following:

1. Creates a three-class, risk-based classification system for all medical devices. Class I devices have minimal safety risks, Class II potential risks, and Class III significant risks.
2. Establishes the regulatory pathways for new medical devices, defined as devices that were not on the market prior to May 28, 1976. Allows devices to get Food and Drug Administration approval and come to market through a new program called 510(k). Under the 510(k) program, Class II devices that are substantially equivalent to devices already on the market received a shortened review by the US Food and Drug Adminis-

tration (FDA). The 510(k) program is a loophole that allows potentially harmful products to come to market.

3. Requires post-market monitoring, including registration and listing of devices with the FDA, good manufacturing practices, and reporting of adverse events involving medical devices.
4. Authorizes the FDA to ban devices that are unsafe.

1990: Safe Medical Devices Act. The intent of this law is to improve post-market surveillance of devices. A 1988 report by the GAO to Congress identified several safety issues related to devices, despite regulatory requirements of the Medical Device Act of 1976.

1. Requires user facilities such as hospitals and nursing homes to report adverse events involving medical devices.
2. Authorizes the FDA to require manufacturers to perform post-market surveillance on permanently implanted devices if permanent harm or death could result from device failure.
3. Defines how a new device can be considered substantial equivalence, the standard for marketing a device through the 510(k) program. Although included in the Safe Medical Devices Act, the 510(k) substantial equivalent category was actually a loophole resulting in the marketing of devices without rigorous testing, resulting in pain, suffering, and death in some patients. This will be discussed later in this chapter.

2010: Affordable Care Act. The ACA (or Obamacare) contained a provision to levy a 2.3% tax on implantable medical devices, to help offset some of the costs associated with the ACA. This tax became effective in 2013 and was operational through 2015. In 2016, Congress suspended the tax for two years, and then in 2018, it was suspended until 2020. The tax was finally repealed in December 2019, as part of a federal spending bill. The device industry has spent millions of dollars on lobbying and campaign contributions on suspension, delay, and repeal measures.

2012: The Food and Drug Administration Safety and Innovations Act. This law touches many aspects of health care, including devices, drugs, and children. While the intent may have been to increase device safety, this act actually watered down some safety requirements. For example, it creates a direct new device pathway, permitting the classification of novel, low-to-moderate risk devices into Class I (lowest risk) or II (rather than Class III) without first having to submit a 510(k). It also places restrictions on early rejection of devices by the FDA.

2016: 21st Century Cures Act. This act was popular among many members of Congress because it provided $4.8 billion to the National Institutes of Health (NIH) for biomedical research. That's a good thing. But the law also watered down the FDA's ability to regulate devices. The medical device industry and others heavily lobbied the FDA. This legislation favored business marketing over patient safety. Elements relevant to devices include the following:

1. Mandates the creation or revision of policies and processes intended to speed patient access to new medical devices.
2. Codifies into law the FDA's expedited review program for breakthrough devices.
3. Expands the application of the "least burdensome" principles in premarket reviews, in other words allowing shortcuts in the review process.
4. Streamlines the processes for exempting devices from the premarket notification 510(k) requirement.

Common Implantable Devices

The list of FDA-approved implantable medical devices covers dozens of pages. Nine of the most common types are reviewed here. I have listed the acquisition price paid by hospitals, freestanding surgery centers, and physician offices. Listed prices vary widely, depending on the brand of device, subtype, and negotiated contract price. The negotiated price is often not disclosed to the public. Prices listed below are therefore given as estimated ranges that a surgery center or hospital pays. The actual charge for the device to patients by hospitals is usually much higher, as much as two to three times the wholesale cost.

Within each category of device are multiple brands, multiple sub-types, and different designs containing different materials. Hip implants can be made as metal-on-polyethylene, ceramic-on-polyethylene, ceramic-on-ceramic, ceramic-on-metal, and, in the past, metal-on-metal. Each metal can contain different mixtures of elements, such as titanium, steel, cobalt, or chromium.

Artificial eye lenses. Many older adults develop cataracts, which simply defined is a cloudy lens in one or both of their eyes. The cloudiness, or opacity, obscures vision leading to loss of vision. When the natural lens is surgically removed, it is replaced with an artificial one. Device cost: $150 to $1,000 per lens. Number implanted: 2,500,000/year.

Coronary artery stents. I have cared for many people who have had coronary artery stents placed in their heart. Most do very well and are able to engage in physical activities that were intolerable before the device was implanted. Coronary arteries provide the blood the heart needs to function. Arteries narrow when they are clogged with plaques containing layers of fat and calcium. An intervention first applied to increase blood flow was to "bypass" the clogged part (called stenosis) with a piece of vein taken from the leg and sewed into the coronary artery. This is a big operation. An easier means of restoring blood flow in the stenotic part of the artery was to insert a metal "spring" that would push open the narrowed artery. This metal spring is very small, less than an inch long and a fraction of an inch in diameter, containing a couple of dollars' worth of basic metal. Device cost for bare metal: $500 to $1,000 each. Drug-coated to help prevent clotting: $1,000 to $2,000 each. Number implanted: 600,000 procedures per year, some with multiple stents ≥1 million a year.

Artificial knees. Artificial knees have brought new life to many people. Knee implants are common, and many of my patients who had severe pain or difficulty walking are now pain free and able to ambulate. In many cases, progressive osteoarthritis has contributed to knee problems, but a long list of reasons for knee replacement exists. People who experience daily severe pain can be made pain free. People who could not walk or who had to use crutches can now walk independently. Device cost: $3,400 to $10,800. Number implanted: 550,000 a year.

Artificial hips. Similar to knees, osteoarthritis and other conditions can result in severe pain and disability. Searing pain can keep patients awake all night. Patients who were unable to walk up a flight of stairs are now able to skip up the stairs. Replacement of a damaged or worn-out hip can be life changing for many people. Device cost: $4,000 to $10,000. Number implanted: more than 250,000 a year.

Orthopedic fracture repair hardware. I'm not an orthopedic surgeon but have talked to surgeons every shift I worked as an emergency department physician. Every day I cared for patients with fractures, and many were admitted to the hospital. Surgeons would take patients to the operating room for ORIF (open reduction and internal fixation). The fixation part requires "nuts and bolts"—fancy screws, metal plates, and other hardware. That's why millions are used each year. Device costs (hardware): A very wide range, with a high mark up by hospitals. For example, NPR News reported that one woman was charged $15,076 for four tiny screws used in her foot (Szabo 2018). Number implanted: >1 million a year (estimated procedures 450,000).

Intrauterine devices. The concept of an intrauterine device as a method of birth control was discussed in the scientific literature nearly 100 years ago; it was not until the 1960s that widespread use occurred. Over the past 50 years, dozens of brands have been marketed. Major brands on the current market fall into two basic types: copper coated and hormone coated. Device cost: $500 to $1,000. Number implanted: 450,000 a year.

Breast implants. Breast implants were developed in the 1960s. Widespread use began in the 1970s. The majority of implants are for cosmetic purposes. Smaller numbers are used in reconstruction after breast cancer removal. Silicone implants are more costly than saline. Device cost: $500 to $2,000. Number implanted: >600,000 a year.

Cardiac pacemakers. Many of the patients I cared for during my career have had implanted pacemakers. There are many types, but the most basic will (1), stimulate the heart to beat, if the heart stops beating, or (2) stimulate the heart to beat if the natural heart beat is too slow to sustain active life. Device cost: $4,000 to $10,000. Number implanted: 240,000 a year.

Surgical mesh. Surgical meshes are a plastic type of mesh, in some cases resembling your screen door. Developed 100 years ago for use in hernia surgery, meshes have seen expanded applications recently, including gynecologic and urologic applications. There are 70 types of meshes on the market. Most patients do well, but there have been problems as described later in this chapter. Device cost: from $100 to >$500, depending on the type. Number implanted: >500,000 a year.

The Economics of Implantable Devices

The device industry is highly profitable. Production costs may only be 10% of the wholesale marketing price. A hip joint that costs less than $400 to manufacture may be sold to a hospital for $4,000. Medtronic, Johnson & Johnson, and Stryker each have over $10 billion a year in global device sales. Corporations can gain an exclusive monopoly on certain devices, eliminate competition, charge outrageous prices, and make enormous profits. Furthermore, minor tweaks can be made to an existing product that results in new patent protections.

Hospitals may also tack on a huge mark up, often two or three times the acquisition cost, and in extreme cases more. That hip joint that cost the hospital $4,000 may be billed out to the patient (or their insurance) for $12,000 or more.

Safety Problems with Implantable Devices

Over the past 20 years, the news media have published repeated stories of problems related to implanted devices. Injury and deaths have been attributed to implants. Legal firms have advertised their services. A paragraph taken from the Riley and Jackson Law Firm (Birmingham, Alabama) website in February 2020 stated, "The medical devices that have harmed our clients include surgical robots, hip implants, knee implants, shoulder implants, IVC filters, transvaginal mesh, hernia mesh, drug coated stents, operating room patient heaters, pacemakers, infusion pumps, and many others."

Brief summaries of some of the most commonly discussed problems follow. *The Bleeding Edge,* a 2018 Netflix documentary that graphically illustrates the safety problems with implanted devices, is worth seeing.

Breast implants. The debate over the safety of breast implants serves as an example of the complex interaction between the courtroom judgments and science. In 1994, a $3.4 billion settlement was paid out in a class action lawsuit involving more than 100,000 women who had become ill after receiving silicone breast implants. Yet the health effects of breast implants are still debated in the scientific literature. The index of peer-reviewed scientific articles, PUB-Med NIH, listed over 3,700 articles as of early 2020 on the topic of "Breast Implant Side Effects." In 2011, the FDA published a summary on the safety of FDA-approved, gel-filled breast implants and updated this in 2018.

Hip devices: traditional metal-on-plastic or metal-on-ceramic. Mechanical failure of artificial hips has been reported, and certain brands of hips have been recalled. It is difficult to determine how many have failed because of design or material problems. However, major law firms have filed lawsuits based on mechanical failure of hip implants.

Hip devices: metal-on-metal. New metal-on-metal ball-and-socket hip devices were introduced in 2000. By 2010, it became apparent that these hips could disintegrate, releasing toxic metal ions, such as cobalt, into the bloodstream, causing cobalt toxicity. The failure rate over five years was 6%, much higher than the traditional metal-on-plastic joints. In 2013, Johnson & Johnson agreed to pay $2.5 billion to settle lawsuits related to its metal-on-metal hip implants.

Mesh problems. Transvaginal mesh was introduced to improve surgical outcomes in women with pelvic organ prolapse and stress incontinence. Unfortunately, the mesh can migrate and push into adjacent structures, causing severe pain. It is sometimes very difficult to remove because of extensive scar tissue. Nearly 100,000 lawsuits have been filed in the United States as a result of transvaginal mesh problems.

Pacemakers. If a pacemaker fails, the heart may stop, and the person may die. Obviously, top safety standards are critical with pacemakers. But there are problems. In 2016, the FDA issued a recall order on over 400,000 pacemakers.

Fixing the Medical Device Safety Problem

As with many problems in the corporate practice of medicine, only the US Congress has the power through legislation to fix the problems associated with the device industry.

1. Require enhanced research and testing before permitting FDA approval of any device.
2. End the 510(k) program and require "substantially similar" products to undergo a rigorous review process.
3. Provide additional power to the FDA to directly inspect and supervise the manufacturing process of devices.
4. Limit patent times to encourage market competition by multiple companies.
5. End the granting of new patents for minor tweaks to devices already on the market and in use.
6. As with other segments of the health care industry prohibit lobbying by the implant device industry and ban contributions to Congressional election campaigns.

Bottom line: The US Congress is overly influenced by device industry lobbyists and campaign contributions that result in weak laws and regulations needed to protect people from potential harmful effects of medical devices.

NINE

Tests and Studies

Radiology, Laboratory, and Technical Procedures

KEY CONCEPTS

1. Busy frontline physicians frequently order thousands of dollars in testing each workday.
2. Many physicians are unaware how much testing costs their patients and health plans.
3. Not all testing, diagnostic, and preventative procedures are needed.
4. Corporate entities make huge profits from physicians ordering tests and studies.

The American College of Radiology spent $3.2 million on lobbying in 2018.
The American College of Pathologists spent $1.3 million on lobbying in 2018.
Quest Diagnostics spent $1.8 million on lobbying in 2018.

When I first began practicing medicine, I never thought twice about the cost of laboratory testing, x-rays, and technical procedures. We were all taught in medical school and residency training programs to order whatever studies we could think of to provide the best care to our patients. We did not want to miss any diagnosis or serious medical condition. In fact, the culture was such that only "dumb doctors" would limit the number of tests compared to "smart doctors." Saving money was not a legitimate excuse. Perhaps the so-called dumb doctors are really the smart ones.

Sadly, in the era of bankrupting health care costs, little has changed. The most vivid examples that stand out in my mind are from bedside rounds in the hospital or emergency department (ED). Bedside rounds are real-time discussions among multiple doctors discussing patient care, laboratory testing, and radiology imaging, usually in front of the patient. Young doctors who can think of ordering the most testing are considered very bright and get glowing evaluations. We even have a name for going overboard and ordering very unusual tests: *serum porcelain levels*. These studies are usually negative. Few, if any doctors give any thought to the cost of any test they order or to who is making a profit when they order lots of testing. Part of this mentality is a result of being lost in the past when testing was relatively inexpensive, and most insurance covered the costs of testing. In addition, 30 years ago, the number of tests available to order fit on just a half-page of paper. Now the number of different tests available has vastly expanded, filling many computer pages. Few doctors have thought to ask what is the price of these new tests. And finding the cost of a test can be nearly impossible. On many occasions, I have attempted to find out the price of a test and spent hours on the phone coming up empty-handed.

Laboratory testing can be expensive: a $17,500 charge for a urine test for drugs of abuse, described by California Health Line on February 16, 2019. That's outrageous corporate profit based on what the health plan said would be a reasonable cost of about $100. Let me describe a common example from my clinical practice: the patient with a sore throat and fever who comes into the office (or ED) during flu season. A nasal or throat swab is commonly used to collect organisms that cause infection. The swab can be sent to an off-site laboratory or analyzed with bedside testing. I can do the bedside test for strep (streptococcal pharyngitis) myself; it is cheap with results in 10 minutes. Similarly, a bedside rapid flu test provides results in 10 minutes. But many of my colleagues send the swab to an off-site laboratory for more exotic tests, such as a $1,000 DNA-PCR respiratory panel. That test can identify a long list of viruses for which we have no treatment. Add tests like this and all the tests that are frequently ordered in the ED and the cost could amount to thousands of dollars. Many of these tests are unneccessary.

Categories of Testing

Testing and studies can be divided into two basic categories: (1) diagnostic and (2) screening-preventative. Diagnostic studies are just that: they help to figure out the diagnosis of a specific symptom—for example, burning during urination, in which case a sample of urine is sent to the laboratory. Another example is obtaining an x-ray for an injured hand. In contrast, screening—preventative studies—search for hidden problems such as screening for high cholesterol or cancer. If these problems are detected early, they can be treated, leading to a healthier person of longer life. Detecting cancer early on may result in a complete cure, whereas cancer detected in late stages may not be treatable.

Diagnostic Studies

I have relied on diagnostic studies my entire professional career to help me determine the correct diagnosis of an illness or to define the anatomy of a patient's injury. One of the most common studies I ordered was a chest x-ray. I would order a chest x-ray for a patient with a fever, a cough, and shortness of breath. The probability of finding pneumonia was high in someone with those symptoms. Taken together with the history, physical, and blood tests, I could determine whether a person needed hospital admission for pneumonia or could be treated at home with antibiotics. For purposes of discussion, I have divided diagnostic studies in to the categories of radiology, laboratory (lab) chemistry, lab microbiology, and technical procedures.

As an ED doctor most of my life, I have looked at thousands of radiographic images. In the early years of my career, x-rays were developed on film, and we would view the films by placing them on a back-light device nailed to a wall of an exam room, with the patient present. There was something very bedside about viewing an x-ray film next to a patient, and my eyes would go back and forth from film to patient. Then, if in doubt of a finding, or lack of one, I could reexamine the patient in real time.

In busy EDs or hospitals, x-ray films would be placed on movable screens that would rotate around in a circle. For example, I'd walk into an adjoining radiology room next to the ED and see a piece of paper taped to the device that would indicate that screen number 22 has Mr. Jones's chest x-ray. I'd push the bottom, and the machine would rotate through multiple x-ray screens until number 22 appeared, and there was Mr. Jones's x-ray. I could even snatch the film (the radiologist might be unhappy if they found out) and take it to Mr. Jones's bed. Of course, I'd view a lot more than chest x-rays, for I've probably looked at every broken bone in the body and more abdominal films than I can count. Long ago we even did lots of skull films in head trauma before CT scans became available.

Now x-rays are computerized and are viewed on a computer monitor. This is great, as the physician no longer has to physically walk to the radiology department to view the x-ray or have it sent by courier to the office. I would argue that is improved bedside medicine resulting in an increase in efficiency. Hospital-based primary care physicians can also view the x-rays on a computer screen in the exam room next to their patients, and have the opportunity to show the x-ray to their patients.

CT scans and MRIs have revolutionized diagnostic medicine. As physicians, we now have a multidimensional view of almost any part of the body. These types of imaging have made possible the treatment of stroke with clot-busting drugs and saved lives of car crash victims who have ruptured internal organs or arteries. Although the machines that perform CT scans and MRIs are expensive, costs of performing individualized tests are affordable considering these machines perform thousands of tests in a year. But here is where the Wall Street business model has surfaced—charges can be outrageous! Charges for many MRI scans done at US hospitals are in the $2,000 ballpark. Compare this to Japan, where similar MRIs are done for $200. That's lots of profit for American hospitals, and we are all paying directly or indirectly.

Before leaving this section on radiology, keep in mind that prices vary widely, even within a given geographic area. I worked at a clinic where the local hospital charged $400 for a chest x-ray. Many of my patients preferred to drive 90 miles round trip to an imaging center that charged only $80 for the same x-ray. And I would get better service at the distant imaging center: the "$80 radiologist" at the distant imaging center would call me the same day and discuss the results. Getting the results from the hospital was frustrating and wasted much of my time because my phone calls were answered by a series of robotic answering machines, phone trees, and long holds. *Bedside medicine* was practiced at the freestanding, $80 x-ray imaging center; in contrast, *corporate medicine* was practiced by that hospital with high prices and bad service.

Blood tests are an important component of diagnostic medicine. Examples of blood tests include

1. Complete blood count: a measurement of red and white blood cells. This test can detect anemia infections, and other conditions.
2. Chemistry panels: electrolytes such as sodium and potassium are measured to assess the functions of the kidneys, the liver, and other organs.
3. Thyroid function tests: tell how well the thyroid gland is working.
4. Lipid panels: can detect elevated cholesterol and other lipid abnormalities.

There are dozens of other tests, including cancer markers, blood-clotting measures, heart attack indicators, and sepsis markers, that would fill this page.

When I started clinical practice, the treating physician could do many of the basic laboratory tests. I have spent more hours than I can count looking into a microscope. Why was this important? This is because a trained human eye can pick up subtle abnormalities that a machine cannot detect. Many times, noticing odd white cells under a microscope was critical in making the correct diagnosis. I would draw blood from a patient's artery for analysis of the arterial blood gas. I would even run the test myself at a machine near the bedside.

As a physician it is frustrating not to know what a patient will be charged for blood tests. It is important to patients because some pay cash and others have to pay a $7,000 out-of-pocket deductible for tests. Different laboratories charge different prices, and one can spend hours on the phone to get a lab to divulge their prices before a test is done only to wind up empty-handed. Likewise, hospitals tend to keep this information secret. Even worse, some hospitals charge extra if the blood tests are drawn in the ED. The exact same test done on the same machine can cost three times more if it originates from the ED because patients are a captive audience.

Microbiology tests are done to identify microorganisms such as bacteria, virus, fungus, or protozoa and are taken from samples from many areas of the body, including urine, stool, spinal fluid, swabs of the nose and throat, draining abscesses, and others. Most commonly involves urine samples but can include pus from an abscess, sputum from the lung, or in cases of very sick patients, organisms found in the blood (sepsis), or spinal fluid. When I began my career, physicians would examine urine and body fluid samples under a microscope, searching for the bad bugs, which would help in choosing the proper antibiotic. There was something special about this basic bedside approach, one trusted the results more than what is now spit out on a computer screen. And when the treating physician does the test the answer is immediate, and directed treatment can start immediately.

To diagnose some diseases, more specialized tests need to be done and are beyond the scope of the average doctor to do at the bedside. Blood samples may need to be taken to determine antibody titers. Antibody titers can help determine the stage of a disease process. Treating a disease in the initial stages may be different compared to when the disease has progressed to late stages. In the past, the presence of antibodies could be determined at the bedside with simple equipment, but now they are done on expensive machines. Like blood chemistry, determining the costs and actual billed charge for these tests is difficult.

DNA Testing

DNA testing is a rapidly advancing field. In 2000, I took a one-year sabbatical to study in an infectious diseases research lab where we did DNA testing to identify bacteria, referred to scientifically as PCR. This was very labor intensive and involved over 60 steps; any error in any step could void the results. Within a few years, machines were designed to take over nearly all the steps. I was involved in the development of a prototype machine as a research project with Lawrence Livermore National Laboratory in California. The analytic machine could do all the 60 steps automatically. Our goal was to identify an organism that caused an illness in a sick person in a matter of 30–45 minutes. We placed our test machine in the ED at UC Davis and would obtain a sample from persons who appeared ill with a high fever. Once we obtained a sample of a person's nasal secretions from their nose, we placed it in the analyzing machine, which would print out a diagnosis after a time period. Our machine was too slow and difficult to operate in the ED environment, but researchers at other institutions were successful in making a rapid diagnosis machine.

Since then, the science and technology of using PCR to identify bacteria and viruses has exploded. Over the years, these machines have become smaller and faster, and they can now match the DNA or RNA fingerprint with nearly every infectious disease agent (germ) known to medical science. Laboratory charges for DNA (and RNA) tests can be high; a commercial respiratory pathogens panel (tests for 10 types of throat/lung infections) can cost over $1,000, much of which is corporate profit. Charges for the same type of testing using PCR technology in Europe are a fraction of the price compared with retail charges in America.

Technical Procedures

Technical procedures using new tools have also exploded in numbers and types during my career. When I attended medical school, the procedures were limited: they included lumbar punctures (to collect spinal fluid and look for meningitis), liver biopsies, and aspiration of abdominal fluid. There was even a major surgery called exploratory laparotomy, which opened up the abdominal cavity to determine the cause of complex abdominal pain.

Now we have a long list of diagnostic procedures, including endoscopy, colonoscopy, bronchoscopy, and many specialized ENT, urologic, and gynecologic procedures. Many of these use flexible fiber-optic scopes. This technology allows the doctor to visualize internal organs, such as the stomach, colon, throat, and lungs. Abnormalities can be identified. Arterial catherization is a procedure in which a tube is introduced into a blood vessel with x-rays taken as a marker dye is injected into a patient. A common example is heart catherization performed by cardiologists to detect abnormalities of heart function and coronary arteries. Cardiac angiography is performed by passing a small tube through a femoral vein and threading it to the heart and has saved thousands from having a full heart attack. Radiology specialists catheterize many types of blood vessels to diagnose abnormalities. New surgery techniques are performed by just poking small holes through a person's skin, such as laparoscopic surgery to remove a gall bladder.

A compassionate doctor will discuss the reasons to do these procedures and risks, exemplifying hands-on bedside medicine. But professional fees charged to patients for many of these procedures are too high and in some cases are flat-out unaffordable. In addition, facility use fees charged by hospitals and surgical centers are exorbitant, with the patient absorbing most of the cost. These fees provide profits for the corporation. Keep in mind that the same procedures are performed in Europe where health care costs are half that of America's.

Overtesting

Ordering an x-ray of the wrist deformed from an injury is a no-brainer. But how many tests should be ordered for someone with vague abdominal pain? Sometimes lost in the discussion are the following questions: How many tests or procedures must be done to save or extend life? How many dollars should be spent on testing to save or extend a person's life? Will the test result in harm?

One example concerns the ordering of head CT scans for minor head trauma in children. The risk of developing cancer after a head CT in young children increases, but by how much is unclear. Is it worth doing 10,000 head CT scans to find one brain injury requiring neurosurgery intervention, when that many CT scans will result in two children developing excess cancers later in life? These questions address philosophical issues, something for medical ethics experts to debate, and is beyond the scope of this book. Research into how to decrease the number of head CT scans for children with minor head trauma is ongoing. Overtesting across the field of health care has generated dozens of scientific articles in 2019 alone.

Screening and Preventative Studies and Procedures

The purpose of screening—preventative studies—is just that: to prevent the development of a serious illness later on. As noted earlier in this chapter, diagnose cancer early and it might be treatable. Diagnosed late, cancer may not be curable. Identifying and treating high cholesterol or other lipids early in life can extend life. Medicare has a long list of preventative tests and procedures. A few examples include:

1. DEXA bone scan (for osteoporosis, a medical term for thin bones)
2. Low-dose lung CT scan (for cancer screening)
3. Diabetic screening (fasting serum glucose and or A1c)
4. Hepatitis C screening
5. Selective abdominal ultrasound (for aortic aneurism)
6. Human immunodeficiency virus (HIV) testing

The Colonoscopy

"Hey, Doc, I got my colonoscopy done yesterday," yelled one of my patients to me as I was picking up some apples in the produce section of my small-town supermarket. So common is this procedure that it has shed any embarrassment. Colonoscopies are now routine screening for the early detection of bowel cancer. Early on, guidelines encouraged persons to have a colonoscopy every 5 years after age 50. This changed to every 10 years, unless a person has a polyp, or other risk factors. Hospitals, surgery centers, and gastroenterologists benefit from revenues generated by performing over 15 million colonoscopies each year. Charges for colonoscopies can be as much as $5,000 to $10,000, although the actual cost to provide the service is less than $1,000. In 2015, Medicare paid $815 for a screening colonoscopy, which includes facility use fee, professional fees, anesthesia, drugs, and other expenses. In other countries, colonoscopies can be done for $500 to $1,000. Some experts argue that better advanced selective screening or doing a limited study called a sigmoidoscopy, which could be done by a bedside primary care physician, would result in fewer colonoscopies. Still others argue that a fecal occult blood test (very cheap) or stool sent to a laboratory for analysis of cancer markers (for example, Cologuard) at $350 would be more cost-effective. New blood tests are also in the pipeline. Will fewer colonoscopies be performed in the future? Only time will tell.

Kidney Dialysis

Kidney dialysis is a technical procedure and does not fall into the classic definition of either diagnostic or screening-preventative test. I have cared for thousands of patients who have kidney failure during many years of medical practice. Each ED shift I worked, three or four patients would come in with problems related to dialysis or kidney failure. In the case of total kidney failure, death may occur in about a week, unless a person receives dialysis or a new kidney transplant. Dialysis is done about three times a week and involves sucking the blood out of a person into a dialysis machine, filtering out the naturally occurring toxins, and then returning the blood to the person. It takes several hours. About a half-million Americans are on dialysis three times a week.

In its infancy, dialysis was performed primarily at university hospitals, but soon independent, privately owned dialysis centers evolved, and dialysis became a business. Dialysis treatment centers have been bought and consolidated by corporations that make enormous profits. In July 2019, *Kaiser Health News* reported on a $524,000 bill sent to a patient who had 14 weeks of dialysis—$13,867 for each dialysis session. However, the Medicare rate is $235 per dialysis session in the area where the patient lives! Fresenius Medical Care, a dialysis company with 2,400 treatment centers, trades on the New York Stock Exchange (FMS). The company canceled the patient's charge after the negative press became national news.

The importance of maintaining high profit margins is further illustrated by actions of the dialysis company DaVita (NYSE-DVA). In the 2018 election cycle, Proposition 8 was placed on the ballot in California. Proposition 8 would limit profit to 115% of the actual costs to run dialysis clinics. DaVita spent over $100 million to get the measure defeated, according to California news media. I was angered by the many TV political ads paid for by DaVita. The TV ads did not present the true facts. California TV viewers were so saturated with the ads, that it was no surprise that Proposition 8 was defeated.

Solutions to the High Costs of Laboratory Tests and Procedures

1. *Post prices.* Congress should pass legislation that requires posting of the full retail prices in understandable language to patients.
2. *Disclose actual costs.* Prior to any tests or procedure, the full price and out-of-pocket price must be provided to patients, and patients must approve.
3. *Ensure physicians' quick review of lab results.* Treating physicians should have the ability to see the actual x-ray or imaging they ordered as soon as the study has been done. The technology exists.
4. *Provide basic bedside bench laboratory facilities.* Physicians should be able to examine their patients' samples under the microscope and perform basic tests in their clinics and hospitals.
5. *Make this industry competitive.* Break up monopolies that currently exist in segments of testing; if that is not feasible, regulate the prices charged.

Bottom line: Many radiology studies, laboratory tests, and technical procedures come with very high prices designed to profit corporate institutions. Like other segments of the health care industry, Congress must stop listening to one sided corporate lobbyists, stop accepting their campaign contributions, and start listening to ordinary Americans.

[TEN]

Nursing Homes and Special Facilities

KEY CONCEPTS

1. As the population ages, the demand for nursing home care increases.
2. The quality of care provided ranges from excellent to atrocious.
3. Corporations are buying and consolidating nursing homes.
4. Agencies that "police" nursing homes may lack the power to improve care.

Nursing homes and their associations lobby Congress, and donate to political campaigns, but precise data are lacking on the total dollars spent in this effort. The American Health Care Association, which represents nursing facilities, spent nearly $4 million each year 2015–2019, nearly $20 million over 5 years, lobbying Congress.

As I write this chapter, one of my patients complained to me about his recent experience at a skilled nursing facility (SNF). "What a racket," he said. "All they want to do is snow you with medications and take your money." He was placed in an SNF for 40 days following an injury from a car crash that resulted in a temporary inability to walk and care for himself. Before going to the SNF, he was on three prescription medications. At discharge from the SNF, he was on 30 prescription medications. On our first visit following his discharge, I took him off 15 medications and discussed tapering off another 10 over the next few weeks.

The definition of a nursing home depends on whom you talk to. This includes a wide range of facilities that offer everything from assisted living, short-term intermediate care, and rehabilitation to long-term permanent care. This chapter will discuss long-term SNFs, which I have personally had the most interaction with during my career. SNFs differ widely in terms of comfort, staff-to-patient ratios, quality of care, cleanliness, food quality, and training and skill of nursing staff.

I have seen the top of the pyramid—the luxury SNFs. In these facilities, patients have private rooms, their own private bathroom, and easy and frequent access to physicians. The nursing staff-to-patient ratio is favorable so that prompt and attentive care is provided, medication errors are minimal, and communication with family members is facilitated by the SNF. Floors, walls, and bathrooms are clean, circulating fresh air, and the food served is wholesome and compares in taste to good restaurants. These facilities are expensive.

I have also set foot in lower-quality SNFs. I recall visiting a distant relative at one of these. I had no sooner walked through the front door and a noxious odor of urine and other foul smells hit me in the face. Two, three, and sometimes even four patients were squeezed into a room. The single bathroom that served each crowded room for four older persons was so dirty I did not want to use it. Messy food trays hung over each bed and the patients seemed to just stare into space. Is this really the way we want our older folks to pass away? Many have helped build America during their lifetimes as machinists, construction workers, engineers, teachers, and nurses. Did we as a nation lose our sense of dignity?

I have also cared for many patients from these not-so-nice SNFs while working in the emergency department. Some patients are brought in with fevers and have pneumonia or a kidney infection. One might think these problems are normal for older bedridden persons, but the evidence is otherwise. An article in *Kaiser Health News* from December 22, 2017, describes the lack of basic hygiene measures in many SNFs that contribute to infections. Still others have fallen from the bed, a chair, or while standing, and arrive in the ED in an ambulance with newly broken bones. We admitted most of the folks who had broken bones, commonly a hip that needed surgery.

But, sadly, this is not all I see. Some patients are sent to EDs because they develop bedsores so deep that bone is exposed; they have not been cared for properly. Other people are so severely dehydrated that they are approaching kidney failure. Why are they dehydrated? In my opinion, because of neglect. I visited a nursing home where food and water trays were removed full and untouched. I looked at a nursing note of an older woman resident, and it said, "Refused dinner." Really? That patient told me she was hungry and thirsty.

On numerous occasions I have reported this type of neglect to state authorities. But it takes several phone calls, long wait times on hold, and sweet persuasion to get someone on the other end of the phone to do something. In the meantime, the ED waiting room is full, and the ED nurse advises me to drop the call because a critical ambulance will arrive in two minutes. There are many other problems with SNFs as described later in this chapter.

The Evolution of SNFs

SNFs provide care for a wide range of conditions. Older persons who are unable to care for themselves occupy many beds, including persons with various stages of dementia, mobility problems (i.e., have difficulty walking), advanced bowel and bladder problems, and, more recently, hospice care patients or those who cannot be at home alone. Younger patients recovering from major injuries or illnesses, brain injury, or advanced forms of neurologic diseases may require the services of nursing homes.

A century ago, many elderly persons were cared for by their adult children in the family home. Cooking, feeding, bathing, and personal care were done by daughters and sometimes sons. Three or even four generations might live under the same roof, and it was expected that in return for mom and dad caring for their young children, the grown-up children would care for their parents when they were no longer independent. Although less common now, in my rural medical practice, I still care for multigenerational families living under the same roof. Grandma and grandpa get good care there.

Over the past 100 years, cultural changes in America have decreased in home care by relatives for several reasons: (1) Women have gone to work, and are no longer at home all day. Even finding daycare for young children can be challenging, and how does one take care of grandma on top of that? (2) Fewer people live in rural areas that provided community support. (3) Complex medication administration adds to the difficulty of caring for the elderly. Grandma in the 1920s most likely took no medications, compared to now when an older person may be on several doses of injected insulin a day and may take 6 to 10 other medications.

That's not to say that every older person in need goes to an SNF. Wealthy individuals can afford to stay in their own homes by hiring help. Visiting nursing, medical assistance, or even home-chore help can be bought for a fee ranging from as few as 4 hours a day to 24 hours a day. Wall Street investment firms have shown interest in this new industry.

The Costs of SNFs

Care in SNFs is expensive. Costs per person for a double room can range from $5,000 to $12,000 a month, depending on the state and even up to $30,000 a month for luxury SNFs. Who pays? Money to pay for SNF care can come from several sources.

Medicare. Medicare provides benefits but only up to 100 days. The first 20 days of care are 100% covered, and then the next 80 days patients also need to pay a co-pay, about $160 a day. Patients must have been hospitalized a minimum of three days as an inpatient. Problems exist when a patient is transferred from a hospital but has been placed under observation. This does not meet Medicare requirements for SNF payments (see section "Observational Status" in chapter 2). What happens if a person still needs SNF care after 100 days? Well, the person then has to dip into any savings. Once a patient's financial resources are depleted, SNFs may assist the person with applying for Medicaid, which will pay for long-term care in certain facilities.

Medicaid. In most states, the Medicaid program will cover the costs of SNFs. But to qualify for Medicaid, persons must be basically "broke." This means spending a person's last dime before getting the program to pay for care. In some cases, older persons have spent their entire life savings for just a few months of SNF care. Some of these persons worked very hard for 40 years and saved every penny they could. To their surprise, and that of their relatives, they may spend their final months or years of life in a filthy room with two or three other once proud Americans.

I have seen families cry. An example stands out in my mind: "Grandpa saved every penny he could, wore shoes until they had holes in them and rarely ate out, and had $48,000 in the bank when he retired. Now you tell me he must give all of this to an SNF for just four months of care?" Yes. Once all his funds are exhausted and he finally has nothing left, Medicaid will pay for SNF care. So many persons have worked hard all their lives, saved, paid off the mortgage, and looked forward to having money for choices during the waning years of their lives. Thirty years of scrimping to save for retirement can all be consumed to pay for the cost of a few months of SNF care.

Private, long-term care insurance. These insurance plans can be purchased but are expensive and may limit coverage. Coverage is usually not forever but for a limited term, for example, one, three, or five years. The amount paid is also capped and could be $100, $150, or $200 a day. A $200-a-day plan is $6,000 per month, a bare minimum to pay for SNFs for most people. Buying a plan when you're young costs less than when you're older. A 55-year-old may pay $2,550 a year for a plan; the same plan would cost over $5,000 a year for a 60-year-old.

Delivering Care in Nursing Homes Is Hard Work

Providing care to residents of SNFs can be challenging. It is hard, almost agonizing. Issues include

1. Dealing with confused patients who may not understand basic instructions
2. Preventing agitated and aggressive patients from disrupting SNF functions
3. Bathing and moving those with mobility problems
4. Taking care of patients with bowel and bladder problems
5. Feeding patients who cannot feed themselves

6. Administering complex medications, sometimes several times a day

7. Recognizing early signs of new illnesses (for example new infections)

Profit versus Nonprofit Business Models

Nursing homes may be owned by for-profit investor groups or families or nonprofit foundations. Nationwide, some 1.6 million people reside in 17,000 nursing homes, and 11,000 of them are for-profit businesses.

The Centers for Medicare and Medicaid Services (CMS) report that nonprofits provide better care than for-profit SNFs. Its analysis found that for-profit chains tend to have (1) a lower staffing-to-patient level, (2) a higher number of deficiencies that could harm patients, (3) higher incidence of pressure sores, and (4) higher hospitalization rates.

The problem with care at for-profit SNFs has been the topic of investigative reporting at major newspapers. Sample story titles from the *New York Times* include: "Care at Nursing Homes Feed Money into Corporate Webs" (Rau 2018) and "At Many Homes More Profit and Less Nursing" (Duhigg 2007).

Problems with Some SNFs

In recent years, the problems with the delivery of care at many SNFs—profits and fees—have been discussed in professional circles, as well as in a series of articles published by leading national and regional media.

The causes of poor quality care are multifactorial and include inadequate staff-to-patient ratios, high turnover of some staff, limited training of some staff, complex patients above skill level of the facility, premature hospital discharge of unstabilized patients, and errors from the requirement to administer too many prescription drugs. As one SNF nurse told me after I called to get details of a patient sent to the ED, "There are just too many very sick people here for the few of us to care for." Poor care results in depression, emotional distress, infections, falls, broken bones, dehydration, pain, malnutrition, and other problems.

Fragmentation of care also contributes to problems for both SNF patients and their staff. Often, SNF patients are not evaluated daily by their attending physicians. There is something to be said about physicians or nurse practitioners who see SNF patients daily and know them well. A call at 1 a.m. by a concerned staff member to the SNF doctor can result in better care than a call to someone who does not know the patient. The latter might result in automatically sending the patient to the ED. In addition, a revolving door of sending a patient from the hospital to the SNF, back to the hospital, and then back to the SNF, all within a few days, results in multiple evaluations by multiple physicians, creating confusion for the patient, redundant testing, and stopping and restarting certain important medications. Too often I have seen patients discharged prematurely from the hospital, only to end up back in the hospital ED a day or two later. That patient was too sick or complex for the level of care the SNF could provide.

Examples of problems in the quality of care provided in some SNFs have been published in the national media. A sample of recommended articles appear next. The article titles provide a flavor of the stories:

1. *Washington Post*: "Overdoses, Bedsores, Broken Bones: What Happened When a Private-Equity Firm Sought to Care for Society's Most Vulnerable" (November 25, 2018); "When Nursing Homes Dump Some Patients to Make More Money" (November 20, 2017).
2. *New York Times*: "Care Suffers as More Nursing Homes Feed into Corporate Webs" (January 2, 2018); "Poor Patient Care at Many Nursing Homes Despite Stricter Oversight" (July 5, 2017); "Facing Lawsuit a Nursing Home in California Seeks Bankruptcy" (February 17, 2015).
3. *Sacramento Bee*: "California's Largest Nursing Home Owner Under Fire from Government Regulators" (June 15, 2015).

4. *Kaiser Health News*: "More Than Half of California's Nursing Homes Balk at Stricter Staffing Rules" (December 7, 2018).
5. National Public Radio Health News: "A Third of Nursing Home Patients Harmed by Their Treatment" (March 5, 2014).
6. *Boston Globe*: "AG Announces Settlements after Allegations That Problems at Nursing Homes Led to Deaths" (March 13, 2019).
7. *Los Angeles Times*: "People Should Be Able to Sue Nursing Homes for Abuse of Elderly Patients, Lawmakers and Activists Say" (August 22, 2017).

The following common issues can be taken from these and other investigative reporting:

1. Some owners of SNFs have put profit ahead of patient well-being.
2. Conditions at some SNFs have harmed patients.
3. Many oversight and policing agencies do not have the resources and clout to enforce regulations.

In addition to the media, several agencies in the US government report on SNFs. CMS has published many reports.

Fraud

There are many examples of alleged fraud within the nursing industry. The extent and types of fraud can be quickly understood by reading a few of the actions published on the US Department of Justice website (https://www.justice.gov/):

1. Kindred Healthcare Inc., have agreed to pay $125 million to resolve a government lawsuit alleging that they violated the False Claims Act by knowingly causing skilled nursing facilities (SNFs) to submit false claims to Medicare for rehabilitation therapy services that were not reasonable, necessary and skilled, or that never occurred, the Department of Justice announced today.

RehabCare Group Inc. and RehabCare Group East Inc. were purchased by the Louisville, Kentucky-based Kindred Healthcare Inc. in 2011 and they now operate under the name RehabCare as a division of Kindred. RehabCare is the largest provider of therapy in the nation, contracting with more than 1,000 SNFs in 44 states to provide rehabilitation therapy to their patients.

2. NASHVILLE, Tenn.—February 5, 2019—Tennessee Health Management, Inc. ("THM") has agreed to pay $9,764,107.98 to settle allegations that it violated the False Claims Act, announced U.S. Attorney Don Cochran for the Middle District of Tennessee. The alleged conduct involved the submission of false claims for payment to TennCare, Tennessee's Medicaid Program, related to nursing facility services to TennCare beneficiaries.

3. The owner of more than 30 Miami-area skilled nursing and assisted living facilities, a hospital administrator and a physician's assistant were charged with conspiracy, obstruction, money laundering and health care fraud in connection with a $1 billion scheme involving numerous Miami-based health care providers.

    "This is the largest single criminal health care fraud case ever brought against individuals by the Department of Justice, and this is further evidence of how successful data-driven law enforcement has been as a tool in the ongoing fight against health care fraud," said Assistant Attorney General Caldwell.

Legal Trickery

Some SNFs require patients to sign away their Eighth Amendment right to file a lawsuit if they are wronged. Instead, they must agree to forced arbitration, in the case of a dispute or bad care that resulted in harm or even death, as illustrated in this *Los Angeles Times* article (Lazarus 2017):

Healthcare, tax reform and the debt ceiling probably will be among the highest-profile issues when Congress returns from a month long recess

Sept. 5. But Democratic lawmakers and consumer advocates already have served notice that they're also going to keep a spotlight on protecting people's right to sue nursing homes for neglect or abuse of elderly patients. The Trump administration, through the Centers for Medicare and Medicaid Services, announced in June its intent to roll back legal rights for consumers put in place under the Obama administration. Those rights include prohibiting any nursing home that receives federal funding—which is most of them—from requiring that disputes be addressed through mandatory arbitration rather than the legal system. Thirty-one senators have written to CMS Administrator Seema Verma during the August recess calling on her to abandon plans to once again allow nursing homes to include mandatory arbitration provisions in their contracts.

Solutions to Problems in Nursing Homes

Many steps can be taken to improve care at nursing facilities. Some solutions include:

1. Federal campaign reform: As with other segments of the health care industry, campaign contributions as well as lobbying by the nursing home industry should be prohibited.
2. Provide regulatory agencies more funding and legal teeth to enforce regulations.
3. Enact legislation at the federal level to better protect SNF patients.
4. Pass federal laws that protect people's right to sue nursing homes for neglect or abuse of elderly patients.
5. Provide funding for daily rounds in SNFs by physicians or nurse practitioners with special training in geriatric care.

Bottom line: Only Congress has the power to enact legislation to correct the problems associated with the corporate intrusion into skilled nursing facilities across America.

Conclusion

This chapter serves to summarize the most important take-home points described in the book. The exam at the end of the conclusion should also help to reinforce major concepts.

Important general concepts described in this book include the following:

1. American health care has slowly evolved from a system of placing patients' well-being first to placing profits first.
2. Health care costs in America exceed $4 trillion a year, over 18% of our gross national product, costing individuals and employers outrageous sums of money.
3. In Western Europe, advanced comprehensive "bedside" health care is provided for half the cost—$6,000 per person per year compared with over $12,000 in the United States.
4. Corporate lobbyists influence US congressional legislative actions or inactions.
5. Independent physicians and single-owner hospitals have consolidated into large systems.
6. National and regional monopolies increase the cost for consumers and business.
7. In-network versus out-of-network health plans can trap and confuse people and result in paying out of pocket for health care.

8. More bedside and less corporate medicine will reduce costs and result in better health care for most people.

9. Federal campaign reform legislation should include a provision that prohibits lobbying and donations by the health care industry.

10. Prices for health care services should be posted in understandable language in the lobbies of hospitals, imaging centers, pharmacies, and physicians' offices, and other providers of health care services.

11. Education of medical students and physicians in residency training programs should include more discussions on fees and charges for medical care.

Take-home points described in specific chapters of this book follow:

Chapter 1. Prescription Drugs

1. Big Pharma has created monopolies for many prescription drugs.

2. Congress has provided "legal loopholes" to allow monopolies.

3. High prices have driven up costs for individuals and insurance companies.

4. Big Pharma's lobbying and campaign donations influence Congress.

Chapter 2. Hospitals

1. In the era of bedside medicine, hospitals served doctors; now doctors serve the hospital.

2. Single stand-alone hospitals have consolidated into large chains creating monopolies that drive up health care costs over the past 30 years.

3. Hospital charges have increased four times or more what they were in the 1980s (adjusted for inflation).

4. Half of the increase in hospital charges result from improved technology and advances in medical care. But the other 50% is unnecessary and results from burdensome regulations,

excessive profits, executive compensation, and administrative inefficiency.

5. Hospital charges may be double or triple the actual costs to provide care and what Medicare determines as fair.

Chapter 3. Physicians

1. Assembly-line corporate protocols have commandeered physicians' independent decisions.
2. Physicians may spend up to 50% of their time on computer data entry, resulting in inefficiency and frustration.
3. Whole bedside health care by primary care physicians has been eclipsed by fragmented care from multiple specialists.
4. Small office-based primary care has given way to hospital-based primary care.
5. Freestanding independent physicians cannot collect a facility use fee; this is a major reason so many practices have been consolidated into hospital systems.

Chapter 4. Health Plans

1. Most US health plans spend only 80% of revenue on actual health care and keep the rest for themselves.
2. In contrast, the US Medicare program and European health insurance plans spend 95–97% of revenue on health care.
3. Health plans frequently limit choice of physicians and hospitals to in-network plans.
4. Use of out-of-network facilities may result in huge out-of pocket costs.
5. Many health plans refuse to pay for needed medical and surgical care.

Chapter 5. European Systems of Health Care Delivery

1. Citizens cannot be denied care for preexisting conditions.
2. Annual individual out-of-pocket expenses are small compared to the United States.

3. Excellent quality of health care is provided at half the US cost.

4. Government agencies regulate and set prices.

5. Europeans are generally happy with their health care systems.

Chapter 6. The Affordable Care Act of 2010 and Other Federal Health Care Laws

1. Federal laws have shaped the delivery of health care in America.

2. The concept of government as a payer for civilian health care started with the Medicare Act of 1965.

3. Many federal laws intent on doing good for the people have loopholes that benefit corporations and increase health care costs.

4. In 2018, over $500 million was spent by the health care industry on lobbying.

5. The Affordable Care Act of 2010 provided protections for many Americans but ushered in increased profits for health plans and other sectors of the health care industry.

Chapter 7. Emergency Departments (EDs)

1. Federal law requires that all people presenting to EDs be evaluated.

2. Overcrowding in EDs results in long waits for minor problems.

3. Corporations exercise increasing control of ED physicians.

4. Hospital charges for care may be very high and may not be covered by health plans.

Chapter 8. The Medical Implant Device Industry

1. Medical device implants are a $300 billion annual industry.

2. Devices have improved the quality of life for many recipients.

3. Most devices have a high profit margin.

4. Safety testing of some devices is lax.

5. Loopholes in device safety laws enacted by Congress have resulted in use of unsafe and harmful devices.

Chapter 9. Tests and Studies: Radiology, Laboratory, and Technical Procedures

    1. Busy frontline physicians frequently order thousands of dollars in testing each workday.

    2. Many physicians are unaware how much testing costs their patients and their health plans.

    3. Not all testing, diagnostic, and preventative procedures are needed.

    4. Corporate entities make huge profits from physicians that order tests and studies.

Chapter 10. Nursing Homes and Special Facilities

    1. As the population ages, the demand for nursing home care increases.

    2. There is a wide range of care provided, from excellent to atrocious.

    3. Corporations are buying and consolidating groups of nursing homes.

    4. Agencies that "police" nursing homes many times lack the power to improve care.

Final Exam

For each question, choose the one best answer.

1. **A key driver of bedside medicine evolving to corporate medicine is**
   a. Consolidation of individual freestanding doctors and hospitals into large groups
   b. The internet and fast computers
   c. Advanced diagnostic technology such as CT scans and MRIs
   d. Medical schools that teach new doctors to follow corporate protocols
2. **Members of Congress have aided the evolution of bedside medicine to corporate medicine because**
   a. Only a few members of Congress (<5%) are doctors
   b. They have ignored the changes

c. Many members have been influenced by corporate lobbyists and accepted campaign donations
   d. They decided corporate medicine provides better health care
3. Current average health care costs in the United States per person per year are about
   a. $500
   b. $4,000
   c. $8,000
   d. $12,000
4. Health care costs in Europe are about half the US costs because
   a. Limitations and price controls on health care fees and charges
   b. European countries deliver inferior care compared to the United States
   c. People die at a younger age in Europe
   d. European hospitals do not have modern CT and MRI scanners
5. Health care corporations make political campaign contributions to members of the US Congress because
   a. It shows that they are patriotic
   b. They receive a tax credit
   c. It might influence how the members of Congress vote
   d. It is a means of disposing of excess capital
6. Some experts claim that US health care costs have increased dramatically over the past 30 years solely because of advances in drugs and technology (e.g., CT scans, cancer drugs, implantable devices). In reality, advances in care have contributed what percent of the rise in costs since 1980?
   a. 100%
   b. 80%
   c. 70%
   d. 50%
7. Admitting patients to the hospital was done primarily by office-based primary care physicians (PCP) in the past. This has evolved to hospital based, in which hospitalists admit most urgent and emergent cases. Reasons for this evolution away from the PCP include

a. Being bogged down with paperwork at the office

b. Increasing hospital requirements and demands to have admitting privileges

c. Decreased payments by insurance companies

d. All of the above

8. **Many health plans have a co-insurance payment obligation. The term *co-insurance* in this context means**

a. People must sign up and pay for a second health plan

b. What a person pays out of pocket, after they reach the deductible amount

c. A person's employer must pay for at least 50% of health plan costs

d. It is the amount a person pays out of pocket for prescription drugs

9. **Medicare health insurance is**

a. Provided free to all children

b. Available to people 65 years old who have paid taxes for at least 10 years

c. Liked by hospitals because payments are higher than private insurance

d. Mostly funded by a 12% payroll tax

10. **Medicaid insurance**

a. Provides the same level of benefits as Medicare

b. Charges individuals between $50 and $100 a month to have this insurance

c. Became more widely available in some states after passage of the Affordable Care Act by Congress

d. Is widely accepted by most all physicians in California

11. **The Affordable Care Act of 2010**

a. Requires everyone to have health care insurance but beginning in 2019 no longer has a penalty for noncompliance

b. Was completely repealed by the US Congress in 2018

c. Limits profit and administrative expense of insurance companies to 12%

d. Was overturned by the US Supreme Court

12. **Regulation of the health care industry in the United States is much less than in Europe because**
    a. Members of Congress are heavily lobbied by the health care industry
    b. European nations are backward in their thinking
    c. Regulation of health care services reduces competition and increases prices
    d. The US Constitution prohibits regulation
13. **Regarding health insurance coverage: a deductible means**
    a. The proportion of money a person may deduct from their income tax
    b. Money deducted from the premium when a person passes a lab test
    c. What people pay out of their pocket before the insurance starts paying
    d. The sum of money deducted from a person's paycheck for health care
14. **Prescription drugs are more expensive in the United States than Europe because**
    a. Federal law has allowed companies to develop a monopoly on many drugs
    b. Most research costs for prototype drugs are paid by the drug companies
    c. Drugs sold in the United States must be made in the United States
    d. The US Food and Drug Administration sets the prices of drugs
15. **Hospital retail prices billed to insurance companies and patients are**
    a. Regulated by state hospital boards
    b. Calculated to be the actual cost of care plus a 10% profit margin
    c. Generally two to three times the actual cost of delivering medical care
    d. Lower in nonprofit hospitals
16. **The insurance industry was able to have a major influence in writing the Affordable Care Act of 2010 because they**
    a. Declared themselves on the side of the American people
    b. Wanted to include the public option

    c. Lobbied Congress and made major campaign contributions

    d. Financed most of President Obama's 2008 campaign for president

17. **Balanced billing**

    a. Means a patient pays the balance between the health plan contribution for care and the full retail fees of the hospital or doctor.

    b. Applies to both in-network and out-of-network fees for services

    c. Is an accounting method used to determine retail fees charged by hospitals

    d. Is forbidden by physicians who work at in-network hospitals

18. **Balanced billing is allowed if patients have the following types of health plans**

    a. Medicare

    b. Medicaid

    c. Private insurance, but receive care by an out-of-network hospital or doctor

    d. All of the above

19. **In-network requirements by health plans**

    a. Limit choice of specialists and hospitals

    b. Expand choice of hospitals but not doctors

    c. Do not apply to primary care doctors

    d. Do not apply if a person goes to an emergency department with an emergency

20. **Federal laws have included language that has helped to increase profits throughout the health care industry because**

    a. It helps to foster a robust market economy

    b. It makes common sense

    c. Profits are invested in future research

    d. Heavy lobbying and campaign donations were made to members of Congress

21. **US health care costs are different compared to Europe because**

    a. We provide better care to everyone

    b. Of the strong dollar compared with the euro

c. We have more advanced drugs, MRIs, and CT scans

d. Of the profit motive among insurance corporations, Big Pharma, hospitals, and others

22. **Medicare Advantage program allows free choice of**

a. Any doctor accepting Medicare

b. Any hospital accepting Medicare

c. Only certain HMO health plans

d. All of the above

23. **Medicare for All has been advocated by some members of Congress. It could lower health care costs because:**

a. It defines the maximum price charged by hospitals, doctors, and others

b. It is already paid for by existing taxes

c. It limits care for those deemed terminally ill

d. It severely restricts surgical procedures

24. **Health plans define in-network doctors and facilities as**

a. Those who have a contract with the health plan, with negotiated fee schedules

b. Those that provide better care

c. Those that meet AACM level 4 or higher health care grades

d. Those where private rooms are paid in full by the health plan

25. **The Emergency Medicine Treatment and Labor Act requires all emergency departments to**

a. Provide free care to persons who are injured in car crashes

b. Have an emergency medicine specialist on duty at least 12 of 24 hours per day

c. Allow transfers to hospitals a with higher level of care after stabilization

d. Provide care by a real medical doctor to every patient who comes to the emergency department

26. **Prescription drug companies may make minor changes to drugs whose patent protection expires because**

a. This allows additional years of exclusive monopoly on the new version of the drug

b. Changes must be done to have these drugs sold over the counter

c. Minor changes to drug delivery (e.g., coated tablet) improve consumers' health

d. It allows for a more efficient means of manufacture

27. **The Affordable Care Act of 2010**

a. Received widespread support from both Democrats and Republicans

b. Prohibits health plans from excluding persons with preexisting conditions

c. Is a short and simple law, a document of only 28 pages

d. Is only effective in states that have also approved the measure

28. **Some prescription drugs have very high retail prices and can cost as much as $700 a pill. The reason prices are so high is**

a. Manufacture of these drugs is costly

b. The drug corporation has a monopoly on specific drugs and can decide on any price they want

c. Drugs are imported and subject to a high tariff

d. They need to recover research and development costs

29. **Hospital retail charges are set by**

a. The government

b. A hospital committee of physicians and attorneys

c. Hospital administrative employees

d. A formula that provides for a 5% profit

30. **The Hatch-Waxman Act of 1986**

a. Provided loopholes that resulted in increased profits for drug companies

b. Repealed the Food, Drug, and Cosmetic Act of 1938

c. Placed a cap on profits by Big Pharma

d. Requires that vaccines first be tested on dogs before being given to humans

31. **A hospital in California charges $100,000 for hip replacement**

a. Medicare will pay only about $33,000 and prohibits balanced billing the patient the remainder of the charge

b. Most health plans would negotiate a low rate in the $40,000–$50,000 range

c. If the hospital is out of network, a patient might be stuck with the full $100,000 bill

d. All of the above

32. The percentage of the US population that has Medicare insurance is

   a. 5%

   b. 15%

   c. 25%

   d. 35%

33. Hospitals may inflate the price of a drug (e.g., cancer drug) or antidote (e.g., rattlesnake antivenin) by three to five times their acquisition (wholesale) price. The main reason hospitals may do this is

   a. This is an easy way to make a big profit

   b. Storage and handling are expensive

   c. The government requires drugs to be stored in a fireproof safe

   d. So a large portion of the profit can be kicked back to the drug company

34. Even with passage of the Affordable Care Act, and paying for health care insurance (having a health plan), a person may lose their home, entire savings, and declare bankruptcy because

   a. The health plan refused to pay for care at an out-of network hospital

   b. The health plan refused to pay for a nonapproved drug

   c. The health plan fails to pay for cancer care

   d. All of the above

35. Nursing homes that fail three inspections by the federal government

   a. Are ordered closed

   b. Face a monetary fine

   c. Must have the owner take a course in improving care

   d. Are taken over by the federal government

36. Regarding nursing homes, individual states may

   a. Impose more stringent regulations

   b. Only inspect those not inspected by the federal government

c. Pass legislation exempting them from federal oversight

d. Mandate that Medicare reimburse the state for unpaid bills

37. **The most common implanted medical device in America is**

    a. Hip implants

    b. Eye lens implants

    c. Breast implants

    d. Heart pacemakers

38. **If a person is cheated by a health plan, hospital, or doctor, they can receive speedy resolution of the problem by**

    a. Filing a criminal complaint with law enforcement

    b. Filing a complaint with the Consumer Finance Protection Bureau

    c. Writing their US congressional representative

    d. There is no speedy resolution. They need to hire a lawyer and file a civil lawsuit.

39. **What action(s) could decrease the cost of health care in the United States?**

    a. Congress could pass laws that place maximum limits on fees and charges

    b. Americans could drink two glasses of alcohol a day

    c. Removing co-pays for doctor visits

    d. All of the above

40. **Some physicians are employed by corporations, also known as practice management groups. One danger of corporations employing physicians is**

    a. There is no danger. This is fake propaganda

    b. Physicians may be ordered to do what is best for the corporations' profit and not what is best for patients

    c. Physicians may become angry and physically attack management

    d. Physicians no longer need to be board certified in their speciality

41. **The electronic medical record**

    a. Has brought medicine from the dark ages to the space age

    b. Has reduced efficiency in many practices

c. Has reduced medical errors

d. Enables doctors to go home early and have free evenings

42. **Individual and small (two or three doctors) freestanding primary care offices have slowly decreased in number because they**

    a. Cannot collect a facility use fee, unlike hospital based–clinics

    b. Attract persons who have no insurance

    c. No longer can collect firewood as payment

    d. Write too many prescriptions

43. **Emergency departments charge a facility use fee to persons receiving care. In larger hospitals, these fees for evaluation of problems like chest or abdominal pain most likely can be**

    a. $50 to $100

    b. $500 to $1,500

    c. $2,000 to $3,000

    d. $3,000 to $6,000

44. **In addition to the facility use fee, emergency departments can also charge fees for**

    a. Medications, both intravenous and oral

    b. Supplies such as bandages and IV tubing

    c. Starting IVs, suturing lacerations, and splinting broken bones

    d. All of the above

45. **Hospitals and doctors' offices generally do not post prices at their facilities because**

    a. Prices change daily

    b. They do not have the personnel to do so

    c. They want to hide their high charges from public view

    d. It is forbidden by law

46. **The HITECH Act of 2009**

    a. Exempts hospitals from lawsuits if they have computerized medical records

    b. Was opposed by the insurance industry

    c. Provided free software that standardized the electronic medical record

    d. Was the driving force behind physicians and hospitals adapting computerized medical records

47. "Meaningful use" as defined by the HITECH Act of 2009
    a. Gives medical professionals wide latitude on type of data entered into the electronic medical record
    b. Requires certain patient information to be entered into the electronic medical record
    c. Prohibits web surfing on medical office computers
    d. Imposes penalties to physicians who enter data that is not "meaningful"
48. The electronic medical record has impacted physicians by
    a. Decreasing efficiency and requiring extra time to input patient data into the computer
    b. Making drawings or sketches of exam findings easier
    c. Increasing overall efficiency
    d. Allowing them to go home early
49. Solo or small primary care group practice has become economically nonsustainable because of
    a. Demands by health plans
    b. Payment schedules that favor hospitals
    c. Electronic medical record requirements
    d. All of the above
50. The most important step to decrease the cost of health care in America is
    a. Discourage consumption of junk food and fast food
    b. Reduce speed limits on highways to 55 miles per hour
    c. Political financial campaign reform that prohibits donations from health care entities to members and candidates of the US Congress
    d. Teaching health care at every grade of K–12 schooling

Answers

1. a	18. c	35. b
2. c	19. a	36. a
3. d	20. d	37. b
4. a	21. d	38. d
5. c	22. c	39. a
6. d	23. a	40. b
7. d	24. a	41. b
8. b	25. c	42. a
9. b	26. a	43. d
10. c	27. b	44. d
11. a	28. b	45. c
12. a	29. c	46. d
13. c	30. a	47. b
14. a	31. d	48. a
15. c	32. b	49. d
16. c	33. a	50. c
17. a	34. d	

If a reference has multiple co-authors, only the first author is listed. This reference list also includes titles of general interest to the reader.

Introduction

Brill S. *America's Bitter Pill: Money, Politics, Backroom Deals, and the Fight to Fix Our Broken Healthcare System.* New York: Random House; 2015.

Callahan D. Cost control—time to get serious. *N Engl J Med.* 2009;361:e10.

CPI Inflation Calculator. US Department Bureau of Labor. https://www.bls.gov/data/inflation_calculator.htm. Accessed April 29, 2020.

The Editorial Board. Make laws, not money. *New York Times.* December 22, 2019.

Fineberg H. A successful and sustainable health system—how to get there from here. *N Engl J Med.* 2012;366(11):1020–1027.

Hoffer E. America's health system is broken: what went wrong and how we can fix it. *Am J Med.* 2019;132(8, pt 3):907–911.

Holly M. How government regulations made healthcare so expensive. Mises Institute Report. May 9, 2017. https://mises.org/wire/how-government-regulations-made-healthcare-so-expensive.

It's time to get mad about the outrageous cost of health care: Why it's so high, how it affects your wallet—and yes, what you can do about it [editorial]. *Consumer Reports.* 2014;79(11):40–48.

Moore M. *Sicko* [Documentary]. Dog Eat Dog Films; 2007.

Ofri D. The business of health care depends on exploiting doctors and nurses. *New York Times.* June 8, 2019.

OpenSecrets. Center for Responsive Politics. Influence & Lobbying/Interest groups. Lobbying and campaign contributions to Congress. www.Opensecrets.org. Accessed April 29, 2020.

Partanen A. The fake freedom of American healthcare. *New York Times.* March 18, 2017.

Rosenthal E. *An American Sickness: How Healthcare Became Big Business and How You Can Take It Back.* New York: Penguin Books; 2018.

Stein J. Congress showers health care industry with multibillion-dollar victory after wagging finger at it for much of 2019. *Washington Post*. December 20, 2019.

Wang P. Sick of confusing medical bills? *Consumer Reports*. April 1, 2018.

Chapter 1. Prescription Drugs

Alpern JD. High cost of generic drugs—implications for patients and policymakers. *N Engl J Med*. 2014;371:1859–1862.

American Association of Retired Persons. The fight to lower prescription drug costs. *AARP Bulletin*. May 2, 2019.

Angell M. *The Truth about the Drug Companies: How They Deceive Us and What to Do about It*. New York: Random House; 2004.

Chen M. Pharmaceutical giants have avoided paying about $2.3 billion in taxes in the US alone. *The Nation*. October 2, 2018.

Dusetzina S. Advancing legislation on drug pricing—is there a path forward? *N Engl J Med*. 2019;381:2081–2083.

Jenkins J. Lowering drug prices. *AARP Bulletin*. October 2019.

Johnson C. The old drug was free. Now it's $109,500 a year. *Washington Post*. December 18, 2017.

Kesselheim A. The high cost of prescription drugs in the United States: Origins and prospects for reform. *JAMA*. 2016;316:858.

Milestones in US food and drug law history. US Food and Drug Administration. https://www.fda.gov/about-fda/fdas-evolving-regulatory-powers/milestones-us -food-and-drug-law-history. Accessed April 29, 2020.

Oliver TR. A political history of Medicare prescription drug coverage. *Milbank Q*. 2004;82(2):283–354.

Pub L No. 98-417. *Hatch-Waxman Act*. Washington, DC: Government Printing Office; 1984.

Rauhala E. As the price of insulin soars, Americans caravan to Canada for lifesaving medicine. *Washington Post*. June 16, 2019.

Richards JR. Droperidol use in the emergency department: Has it changed since the Food and Drug Administration warning? *Ann Emergency Medicine*. 2002;40(4):S60.

Rowland C. Investigation of generic "cartel" expands to 300 drugs. *The Washington Post*. December 9, 2018.

Shesgreen D. Pharma paid patient groups. *USA Today*. February 13, 2018.

Thomas K. A drug costs $272,000 a year. Not so fast, says New York State. *New York Times*. June 24, 2018.

US Department of Justice. GlaxoSmithKline to plead guilty and pay $3 billion to resolve fraud allegations and failure to report safety data. Office of Public Affairs. July 2, 2012.

US Senate. S. Rep. No. 114-429 (2015-16).

Warraich H. A costly PBM trick: Set lower copays for expensive brand-name drugs than for generics. *Stat News*. March 12, 2018. www.statnews.com/2018/03/12.

Chapter 2. Hospitals

Abelson R. Many hospitals charge double or even triple what Medicare would pay. *New York Times*. May 9, 2019.

Anderson C. California AG to challenge Sutter Health pricing practices as anti-trust trial begins Monday. *Sacramento Bee*. September 22, 2019.

Appleby J. Meow-ch! The $48,512 cat bite. Bill of the Month. *Kaiser Health News*. February 27, 2019.

Beaulieu N. Changes in quality of care after hospital mergers and acquisitions. *N Engl J Med*. 2020;382:51.

Bei G. Extreme markup: The 50 hospitals with the highest charge to cost ratio. *Health Affairs*. 2015;34(6). https://doi.org/10.1377/hlthaff.2014.1414.

Brill S. What I Learned From My $190,000 Surgery. *Time*. January 8, 2015.

Eaton J. Hospitals grab at least $1 billion in extra fees for emergency room visits. Public Integrity. September 20, 2012.

Hancock J. UVA has ruined us: Health system sues thousands of patients, seizing paychecks and putting liens on homes. *Washington Post*. September 9, 2019.

Heredia Rodriguez C. Summer bummer: A young camper's $142,938 snakebite. Bill of the Month. *Kaiser Health News*. April 30, 2019.

Hospital executive compensation. *Sacramento Business Journal*. June 27, 2012.

Jameson M. Florida hospital whistleblower case widens to allege billing fraud in emergency departments. *Orlando Sentinel*. October 17, 2012.

Kliff S. Emergency rooms are monopolies: Patients pay the price. Vox. December 4, 2017. https://www.vox.com/health-care/2017/12/4/16679686/emergency-room -facility-fee-monopolies.

Kliff S. With medical bills skyrocketing more hospitals are suing for payment. *New York Times*. November 8, 2019.

Meier B. Hospital billing varies widely government data shows. *New York Times*. May 8, 2013.

Never a bargain. *The Economist*. June 29, 2019.

Ofri D. Nonprofit Hospitals Are Too Profitable. *New York Times*. February 23. 2020.

Richards JR. Patients prefer boarding in inpatient hallways: Correlation with the National Emergency Department Overcrowding Score. *Emerg Med Int*. 2011;2011:840459. http://dx.doi.org/10.1155/2011/840459.

Rosenthal E. The beloved hospital? *New York Times*. September 1, 2019.

Sunshine is a partial disinfectant. *The Economist*. November 23, 2019.

Thomas W. The nonprofit hospital that makes millions, owns a collection agency and relentlessly sues the poor. ProPublica. June 27, 2019.

US Department of Justice. Community Health Systems Inc. to pay $98.15 million to resolve False Claims Act allegations. Office of Public Affairs. August 4, 2014.

US Department of Justice. Hospital chain will pay over $260 million to resolve false billing and kickback allegations; one subsidiary agrees to plead guilty. Office of Public Affairs. September 25, 2018.

US Department of Justice. Hospital chain will pay over $513 million for defrauding the United States and making illegal payments in exchange for patient referrals: Two subsidiaries agree to plead guilty. Office of Public Affairs. October 3, 2016.

US Department of Justice. United States intervenes in False Claims Act lawsuit against Prime Healthcare Services Inc. and its CEO alleging unnecessary inpatient admissions from emergency rooms. Office of Public Affairs. May 25, 2016.

Wong P. Sick of Confusing Medical Bills? *Consumer Reports*. August 1, 2018.

You elected them to write the law. They're letting corporations do it instead. Center for Public Integrity. publicintegrity.org. April 4, 2019.

Chapter 3. Physicians

Axelrod J. Family hit with $3,700 bill for out-of-network anesthesiologist. *CBS News*. April 17, 2019.

Bindman A. Curbing surprise medical bills can be a window into cost control. *JAMA*. 2018;320:2062.

Buchwald H. Courtesy: Professional, patient, personal. *General Surgery News*. April 2019.

Classen D. Finding the meaning in meaningful use. *N Engl J Med*. 2011;365:855.

Cooper Z. Out-of-network emergency-physician bills—an unwelcome surprise. *N Engl J Med*. 2016;375:1915.

Crum B. Former Mercy doctor wins appeal in $1.5 million wrongful termination lawsuit. *Springfield Ledger-News*. January 24, 2018.

Lee B. Doctors wasting over two-thirds of their time doing paperwork. *Forbes*. September 7, 2016.

Lyu H. Overtreatment in the United States. *PLoS One*. September 6, 2017. https://doi.org/10.1371/journal.pone.0181970.

Meigs S. Electronic health record use a bitter pill for many physicians. *Perspect Health Inf Manag*. 2016;13:1d.

Mosley M. No Metric Bonus is Worth Your Soul. *Emergency Medicine News*. April 2020. 42(4):3

Noseworthy J. The future of care—preserving the patient-physician relationship. *N Engl J Med*. 2019;381:2265.

Ofri D. Perchance to think. *New Engl J Med*. 2019;380:1197.

116th US Congress. Stopping the outrageous practice of Surprise Medical Bills Act of 2019. S. 1531. Library of Congress.

Reiter M. Advocacy efforts in support of due process. *Common Sense*. July/August 2015.

Rosenthal E. After surgery, surprise medical bill from a doctor he didn't know. *New York Times*. September 20, 2014.

Sanger-Katz M. Mystery solved: Private-equity-backed firms are behind ad blitz on "surprise billing." *New York Times*. September 13, 2019.

Sanger-Katz M. Senator calls for inquiry into "surprise" medical bills. *New York Times*. December 3, 2016.

Sessums L. Primary care first—is it a step back? *N Engl J Med*. 2019;381:898.

Shopes R. Doctor says she was fired for reporting low staffing levels at Brandon Regional ER. *Tampa Bay Times*. February 20, 2015.

US Department of Justice. Detroit area doctor sentenced to 45 years in prison for providing medically unnecessary chemotherapy to patients. Office of Public Affairs. July 10, 2015.

US Department of Justice. Healthcare service provider to pay $60 million to settle Medicare and Medicaid False Claims Act Allegations. Office of Public Affairs. February 8, 2017.

Wensel R. RVU medicine technology and physician loneliness. *N Engl J Med*. 2019;380:305.

Williams & Jensen PLLC. Permanent doc fix signed into law. *Common Sense*. May/
June 2015.

Wright A. Physician burnout—redesigning care to restore meaning and sanity for
physicians. *N Engl J Med*. 2018;378:309.

Chapter 4. Health Plans

Abelson R. Federal watchdog questions billions of dollars paid to private Medicare
plans. *New York Times*. December 12, 2019.

Bergthold L. Medical necessity: Do we need it? *Health Aff*. 1995;14(4):180–190.
https://doi.org/10.1377/hlthaff.14.4.180.

Christensen J. Fairness, greed, and balanced billing: Insurance companies vs.
everyone. *Common Sense*. March 2016.

Brown E. Stalled federal efforts to end surprise billing—the role of private equity.
N Eng J Med. 2020:382:1189.

Cooper Z. Out-of-network emergency physician bills—an unwelcome surprise.
N Engl J Med. 2016;375:219.

Derlet RW. Commentary: Locked gates, profit and pain. *Acad Emerg Med*.
1997;4:1099.

Derlet RW. The impact of health maintenance organization care authorization policy
on an emergency department before California's new managed care law. *Acad
Emerg Med*. 1996;3:338.

Girouard J. Capitalist case for nonprofit health insurance. *Forbes*. October 12, 2009.

Gruber L. The movement to industry: The growth of HMOs. *Health Aff*. 1988;7(3).
https//doi.org/10.1377/hlthaff.7.7197.

Kronick R. Medicare and HMOs—the search for accountability. *N Engl J Med*.
2009;360:2048.

Penno, LA. *Managed Care Ethics: The Close View Prepared for U.S. House of
Representatives Committee on Commerce Subcommittee on Health and Environment*. May 30, 1996.

Provost C. Medicaid: 35 years of service. *Health Care Financ Rev*. 2000;22:141.

Riner RM. Are usual and customary charges reasonable? *West J Emerg Med*.
2016;17:684.

Rosato D. Patients getting stuck with big bills after ER visits. *Consumer Reports*.
February 9, 2018.

Sanger-Katz M. A health insurer tells patients it won't pay their bills, but then pays
them anyway. *New York Times*. July 19, 2018.

Shaw G. Studies rebut Anthem's retrospective ED denials. *Emergency Medicine
News*. 2019;41:8.

Sottilli C. My elderly mom was treated in the ER, recovered and came home. Then
the surprise medical bills started coming in. *Washington Post*. November 16,
2019.

Terhume C. As billions in tax dollars flow to private Medicaid plans, who's minding
the store? *Kaiser Health News*. October 19, 2018.

Thompson M. Why a patient paid a $285 copay for a $40 drug. *PBS News*.
August 19, 2018.

Valine K. Modesto sues broker it claims connected it with sham health insurer seeks
$8.3M. *Modesto Bee*. June 8, 2019.

Van Nuys K. Frequency and magnitude of co-payments exceeding prescription drug costs. *JAMA*. 2018;319:1045.

Chapter 5: European Systems of Health Care Delivery

Bey TA. The current state of hospital-based emergency medicine in Germany. *Int J Emerg Med*. 2008;1:273.

Chevreul K. France: Health system review. *Health Syst Transit*. 2015;17(3):1–218.

De Pietro C. Switzerland: Health system review. *Health Syst Transit*. 2015;17(4):1–288.

The fix for American care can be found in Europe. *The Economist*. August 10, 2017.

Frayer L. UK hospitals are overburdened, but the British love their universal health care. NPR News. March 7, 2018.

International Health Care Health System Profiles: The Commonwealth Fund. 2019. www.international.commonwealthfund.org.

Kroneman M. Netherlands: Health system review. *Health Syst Transit*. 2016;18(2):1–240.

Lundberg C. $200 minus $200. *Slate*. January 27, 2014.

Minchin M. Quality of care in the United Kingdom after removal of financial initiatives. *N Engl J Med*. 2018;379:948.

Reid TR. *The Healing of America: A Global Quest for Better, Cheaper, and Fairer Health Care*. Waterville, ME: Thorndike Press; 2009.

Stock S. Integrated ambulatory specialist care—Germany's new healthcare sector. *N Engl J Med*. 2015;372:1781.

Struijs J. Integrating care through bundled payments: Lessons from the Netherlands. *N Engl J Med*. 2011;364:990.

Van der Linden C. Emergency department crowding in the Netherlands: Managers' experiences. *Int J Emerg Med*. 2013;6:41.

Van der Linden N. Effects of emergency department crowding on the delivery of timely care in an inner city hospital in the Netherlands. *Eur J Emerg Med*. 2016;23:337.

van Ginneken E. Implementing insurance exchanges—lessons from Europe. *N Engl J Med*. 2012;367:691.

Chapter 6: The Affordable Care Act of 2010 and Other Federal Health Care Laws

Blumenthal D. The Affordable Care Act at 5 years. *N Engl J Med*. 2015;272:2451.

Burde H. The HITECH Act: An overview. Health Law. *AMA J Ethics*. 2011;13:172.

Cohen WJ. Reflections on the enactment of Medicare and Medicaid. *Health Care Financ Rev*. 1985;Suppl:3–11.

Donohue J. Doughnuts and discounts—changes to Medicare Part D under the Bipartisan Budget Act of 2018. *N Engl J Med*. 2018;378:1957.

Dorsey JL. The Health Maintenance Organization Act of 1973 (P.L. 93-222) and prepaid group practice plans. *Med Care*. 1975;13:1.

McGreal C. Revealed: Millions spent by lobby firms fighting Obama health reforms. *The Guardian*. October 1, 2009.

US Public Law 75-717. *Federal Food, Drug, and Cosmetic Act of 1938*. Washington, DC: Government Printing Office; 1938.

US Public Law 89-97. *Social Security Act Amendments of 1965 (Health Insurance for the Aged Act)*. Washington, DC: Government Printing Office; 1965.

US Public Law 104-191. *The Health Insurance Portability and Accountability Act of 1996*. Washington, DC: Government Printing Office; 1996.

US Public Law 108-173. *Medicare Prescription Drug Improvement and Modernization Act of 2003*. Washington, DC: Government Printing Office; 2003.

US Public Law 111-148. *Patient Protection and Affordable Care Act of 2010*. Washington, DC: Government Printing Office; 2010.

Wagner J. Democrats fail to overturn Trump Administration rule on "junk" insurance plans. *The Washington Post*. October 10, 2018.

Zuabi N. Emergency Medicine Transfer and Labor Act: OIG patient dumping settlements. *West J Emerg Med*. 2016;17:245.

Chapter 7. Emergency Departments

AAEM/RSA Advisory Committee. Lay corporations running residency programs. *Common Sense*. March/April 2019.

Ballard D. EMTALA: Two decades later; a descriptive review of fiscal year 2000 violations. *Am J Emerg Med*. 2006;24:197.

Creswell J. The company behind many surprise emergency room bills. *New York Times*. July 24, 2017.

Derlet R. Corporate and hospital profiteering in emergency medicine: Problems of the past, present and future. *J Emerg Med*. 2016;50:902.

Derlet RW. Administrators Should Own Up to EMR Errors. *Emergency Medicine News*. April 2020,42(4):11.

Derlet RW. Emergency department crowding and loss of licensure: A new risk of patient care in hallways. *West J Emerg Med*. 2014;15:137.

Derlet RW. Overcrowding in emergency departments: Teaching, non-teaching hospitals, and state government. *Common Sense*. 2000;7:18.

Derlet RW. Ten solutions for emergency department crowding. *West J of Emerg Med*. 2008;8:137.

Hsia R. Variation in charges of emergency department visits across California. *Ann Emerg Med*. 2014;64:120.

Keaney J. *The Rape of Emergency Medicine*. Phoenix. 1992. ISBN 10: 0963223712.

Kincaid E. Envision healthcare infiltrated America's ERs. Now it's facing a backlash. *Forbes*. May 15, 2018.

McNamara RM. A survey of emergency physicians regarding due process, financial pressures, and the ability to advocate for patients. *J Emerg Med* 45:111–116. 2013.

McNamara R. The corporate practice of emergency medicine. American Academy of Emergency Medicine. 2019. https://www.aaem.org/get-involved/sections/yps/rules -of-the-road/corporate-practice.

Millard W. Nothing to lose but our chains. *Ann Emerg Med*. 2017;69(4):15A–20A.

Richards JR. Patients prefer boarding in inpatient hallways: Correlation with the National Emergency Department Overcrowding Score. *Emerg Int J*. 2011:2011; 840459. htttp://dx.doi.org/10.1155/2011/840459.

Rosenthal E. Where the frauds are all legal. *New York Times*. December 7, 2019.

Rowland C. Why the flight to the hospital is more costly than ever. *Washington Post*. July 1, 2019.

Simons S. Why EMRs don't work for EPs. *Emergency Medicine News*. January 2020,42(1):9.

Sorelle R. Staffing companies hospitals fail to pay EPs. *Emergency Medicine News*. January 2019;41(1):1,34.

US General Accounting Office Report to Congressional Committees. *Emergency care: EMTALA administration and enforcement issues*. GAO-747 EMTALA. June 22, 2001.

Chapter 8. The Medical Implant Device Industry

Dick K. *The Bleeding Edge* [Documentary]. Shark Island Productions; 2018.

Drummond J. Metal-on-metal hip arthroplasty: A review of adverse reactions and patient management. *J Funct Biomater*. 2015;6:486.

Faris O. The changing face of clinical trails: An FDA viewpoint on unique considerations for medical device clinical trials. *N Engl J Med*. 2017;376:350.

Kaplan A. Medical device makers spend millions lobbying to loosen regulations in D.C. *NBC News*. December 3, 2018.

Lenzer J. Can your hip replacement kill you? *New York Times*. January 13, 2018.

Lind K. Understanding the market for implantable medical devices. *Insight on the Issues 129*. AARP Public Policy Institute. August 2017.

Marcus H. Regulatory approval of new medical devices. *BMJ*. 2016;353:i2587.

Mattke S. Medical device innovation in the era of the Affordable Care Act. *Rand Health Q*. 2016;6:9.

Oliver J. Medical devices. *Last Week Tonight with John Oliver*. HBO. June 2, 2019.

Rathi V. Characteristics of clinical studies conducted over the total product life cycle of high-risk therapeutic medical devices receiving FDA premarket approval in 2010 and 2011. *JAMA*. 2015;314:604.

Rising J. Delays and difficulties in assessing metal-on-metal hip implants. *N Engl J Med*. 2012;367:e1.

Szabo l. Sticker shock jolts Oklahoma patient: $15,076 for 4 tiny screws. NPR News. May 18, 2018.

Thompson M. Medical device recalls and transparency in the UK. *BMJ*. 2011;342:d2973.

Valoir T. Patent strategy for medical products: Intellectual property and technology. *Law Journal*. 2011;23:8.

Zuckerman DM. Medical device recalls and the FDA approval process. *Arch Intern Med*. 2011;171:1006.

Chapter 9. Tests and Studies

Cross AJ. Whole-colon investigation vs. flexible sigmoidoscopy. *Br J Cancer*. 2019;120:154.

Gathering the Evidence. *The Economist*. April 27, 2019.

Gold J. They may owe nothing—half million dollar dialysis bill cancelled. Bill of the Month. *Kaiser Health News*. July 26, 2019.

Létant SE. Multiplexed reverse transcriptase PCR assay for identification of viral respiratory pathogens at the point of care. *J Clin Microbiol*. 2007;45:3498.

Maida M. Screening for colorectal cancer: Present and future. *Expert Rev Anticancer Ther*. 2017;17:1131.

Medicare payment schedule for colonoscopies. https://aspe.hhs.gov/system/files/pdf
/255906/DHNAdditionalInfor.pdf.

Nishijima D. Cost-effectiveness of the PECARN rules in children with minor head
trauma. *Ann Emerg Med.* 2015;65:72.

Pliakos EE. The cost-effectiveness of rapid diagnostic testing for diagnosis of
bloodstream infection. *Clin Microbiol Rev.* 2018;31:e00095:17.

Regan J. A sample-in-answer-out instrument for the detection of multiple respiratory
pathogens in unprepared nasopharyngeal swab samples. *Analyst.* 2010;135:2316.

Sanger-Katz M. They want it to be secret: How a common blood test can cost $11 or
almost $1,000. *New York Times.* April 30, 2019.

US Public Law 100-578. *Clinical Laboratory Improvement Amendments of 1988.*
Washington, DC: Government Printing Office; 1988.

Chapter 10. Nursing Homes and Special Facilities

California Health and Safety Code. HSC Section 1267.13.

Comondore V. Quality of care in for-profit and not-for-profit nursing homes: Systemic
review and meta-analysis. *BMJ.* 2009;339:b2732. doi:10.1136/bmj.b2732.

Duhigg C. At many homes more profit and less nursing. *New York Times.* September 23, 2007.

Harrington C. Does investor ownership of nursing homes compromise the quality of
care? *Am J Public Health.* 2001;91:1452.

Jaffe I. A third of nursing home patients harmed by their treatment. *All Things
Reconsidered.* NPR. March 5, 2014.

Lazar K. AG announces settlements after allegations that problems at nursing homes
led to deaths. *Boston Globe.* March 13, 2019.

Lazarus Z. People should be able to sue nursing homes for abuse of elderly patients,
lawmakers and activists say. *Los Angeles Times.* August 22, 2017.

Lundstrom M. California's largest nursing home owner under fire from government
regulators. *Sacramento Bee.* June 15, 2015.

Oslander J. Reducing unnecessary hospitalizations of nursing home residents. *N Engl
J Med.* 2011;365:1165.

Ostrov BF. More than half of California's nursing homes balk at stricter staffing
rules. *Kaiser Health News.* December 7, 2018.

Rau J. Care suffers as more nursing homes feed into corporate webs. *New York
Times.* January 2, 2018.

Rau J. Infection Lapses Rampant in Nursing Homes But Punishment Rare. *Kaiser
Health News.* December 22, 2017.

Rau J. Poor patient care at many nursing homes despite stricter oversight. *New York
Times.* July 5, 2017.

Singletary M. When nursing homes dump some patients to make more money.
Washington Post. November 20, 2017.

Thomas K. Facing lawsuit a nursing home in California seeks bankruptcy. *New York
Times.* February 17, 2015.

US Public Law 100-203. *Omnibus Reconciliation Act of 1987, Nursing Home
Reform.* Washington, DC: Government Printing Office; 1987.

Whoriskey P. Overdoses, bedsores, broken bones: What happened when a private-
equity firm sought to care for society's most vulnerable. *Washington Post.*
November 25, 2018.

medical educational education (CME), 52
medical implant devices, 134–43, 169
medical loss ratio, 75, 110, 114
medical savings accounts, 78
medical school: ED training, 120–21, 126; education on costs, 1–2, 4, 144, 167; requirements, 50; residencies, 47, 50–51, 120–21, 126; training overview, 47, 50–52; tuition, 50, 65
medical staff executive committees, 41, 42
Medicare: and balanced billing, 80; benefits, 80; deductible, 38, 80; and dialysis, 153–54; DRGs, 35, 94, 103, 107; eligibility, 80; fraud, 39–40, 65, 163; gap insurance, 81; legislation on, 10–11, 71, 81, 107, 108–9; medical loss ratio, 67, 89, 168; Medicare for All, 38, 103, 104; and observational status, 42–43, 159; and prescriptions, 10–11, 24, 80, 81, 93, 103, 104, 108–9; as pricing model, 35, 37, 43, 44, 65, 103, 104, 132; and skilled nursing facilities, 159; and testing, 81, 183; tying tuition to, 65; up-coding, 81, 82
Medicare Act of 1965, 105, 107, 169
Medicare Advantage. See Medicare Part C
Medicare Part A, 80
Medicare Part B, 80, 81, 103
Medicare Part C, 73, 80, 81–82
Medicare Part D, 80, 81, 108–9
Medicare Prescription Drug, Improvement, and Modernization Act of 2003, 10–11, 81, 108–9
Merck, 18
meshes, surgical, 141, 142
microbiology tests, 146, 149
MOC (maintenance of board certification), 52
monopolies: drug makers, 6, 7–8, 11–20, 23, 24, 167; health insurers, 88; hospitals, 28, 30, 34, 36, 37, 42, 44, 84, 167; testing, 154
MRIs, 33, 75, 86, 126, 147
Mylan, 8

narcotics, 9–10
National Health Care Institute (Netherlands), 100

National Health Service (NHS), 94, 95–97, 103
National Institutes of Health (NIH), 23, 138
Neidorff, Michael, 69
Netherlands, 100–101, 104
nurse practitioners, 64
nursing homes. See skilled nursing facilities

Obamacare. See Affordable Care Act
observational status, 42–43, 159
Office of Inspector General, 19–20
office visits, 55, 81, 88
Oliver, John, 39
open reduction and internal fixation (ORIF), 140
orphan drugs, 14
orthopedic fracture repair, 140
oseltamivir, 18–19
osteopathic schools, 50
out-of-network. See in-network/out-of-network health care
out-of-pocket charges: annual maximum, 74–75; and employer-based plans, 78; European systems, 91, 94, 96, 97, 99, 100, 102, 168; high costs of, 67, 166, 168; and insurance status, 37–38
overcrowding in EDs, 118–19, 121–22, 124–25, 126, 132, 169

pacemakers, 135, 136, 140–41, 142–43
Pallone, Frank, 22
patents, 8, 23, 24, 108, 136, 143
pathologists, 55, 144
patient's financial bill of rights, 45
PCR. See DNA testing
Peeno, Linda, 72
Pelosi, Nancy, 24
Pfizer, 15–16, 20
Pharmaceutical Research and Manufactures of America (PhRMA), 16–17
pharmaceutical sales representatives, 15–16
pharmacies, 14–15, 85
physician assistants, 64
physician governing body, 31
physician groups, 129–31

About the Author

Dr. Robert W. Derlet served as a member of the School of Medicine faculty at the University of California, Davis, for over 20 years and is currently Professor Emeritus. He also served as a candidate for the US Congress during the November 2016 presidential election. During that election cycle, he spent 18 months campaigning in one of the largest congressional districts in California, the fourth, which spans 300 miles of the Sierra Nevada Foothills, from Lake Tahoe south to Yosemite and Kings Canyon National Parks. Dr. Derlet faced angry crowds at town hall meetings, with so many people expressing their frustrations with our current system of health care delivery, complaining that it has evolved to only benefit pharmaceutical, hospital, and insurance corporations. They were angry with a Congress that they believed does not truly serve the people, but rather too often answers to high-paid lobbyists and the health care corporations that influence many members of the US Congress through political donations.

Dr. Derlet's health care perspective has evolved over 40 years from many avenues in the health care delivery system. This includes personal experience of "hands-on" caring for tens of thousands of patients, beginning in the 1970s and continuing into 2019; research on health care delivery; and teaching in medical schools and colleges. His international perspective has been shaped as a visiting professor in 8 European countries over the years, where he saw firsthand that outstanding medical care can be delivered at half the costs in America.